Contents

Introduction   1
Defining importance of diseases   1
FAO/EMPRES: a new emphasis   2
Early detection   3
The need for surveillance   4
What is surveillance?   4
Surveillance on the ground   5
Putting a surveillance system in place   5
Surveillance for what?   7
Surveillance when and how?   8
Surveillance in resource-poor countries   18
Information systems   20
Setting the goals; determining needs and outputs   23
Computerisation   25
Questionnaire design   31
Databases   34
Data quality control   36
Feedback   39
The role of GIS   40
Motivating and training field staff   42
Awareness creation among decision-makers   43
Using surveillance as a management tool   45
FAO involvement in surveillance and information systems development   46
Examples of questionnaires   48

Appendix: I Random sample design   55
Appendix: II A model framework for strengthening disease surveillance   59

Further reading   71

Acknowledgements

The text for this manual was prepared in FAO by Dr Roger Paskin (Animal Health Officer) and reviewed by the professional staff of the Infectious Diseases Group, Animal Production and Health Division. The contribution of Dr Chris Baldock (Ausvet Consultants) in writing the material for Appendix II is gratefully acknowledged.

MANUAL
ON LIVESTOCK DISEASE
SURVEILLANCE AND
INFORMATION SYSTEMS

FOOD AND AGRICULTURE ORGANIZATION OF THE UNITED NATIONS
Rome, 1999

Reprinted 2003

ISBN 92-5-104331-0

Manual on Livestock Disease Surveillance and Information Systems

Introduction

The FAO has always been concerned with agricultural development and food security. Recent disease epidemics, in both developing and industrialised countries, have once again focussed attention on livestock diseases and their potential to harm development. In the context of developing countries, disease epidemics do four things:

- They reduce herds and flocks dramatically, which, in the case of pastoral peoples, is a major blow to food security and the ability to survive;

- They cause trading partners to – quite understandably – put trade barriers in place in order to protect their own countries from infection. Where livestock or meat exporting countries are affected by epidemics, their "pariah" status can cost millions of dollars in terms of foreign exchange losses, and drive farmers and the local meat industry to the wall.

- They are a deterrent to sustained livestock production.

- They add significantly to the cost of livestock production through the necessity for the application of costly disease control measures.

Defining the importance of diseases

When does a disease become important enough to warrant official intervention? Or to merit international attention? Much attention has been given to highlighting this issue in recent years. The International Office for Epizootics (OIE) has classified animal diseases into two "lists" – List A and List B in order to characterise their level of significance in terms of international trade.

The most important diseases are classified under LIST A. The definition of List A diseases is:

"Transmissible diseases which have the potential for very serious and rapid spread, irrespective of national borders, which are of serious socio-economic or public health consequence and which are of major importance in the international trade of animals and animal products."

List A diseases are:

Foot and mouth disease
Swine vesicular disease
Peste des petits ruminants

Vesicular stomatitis
Rinderpest
Contagious bovine pleuropneumonia

1

Lumpy skin disease   Rift Valley fever
Bluetongue   Sheep pox and goat pox
African horse sickness   African swine fever
Classical swine fever   Highly pathogenic avian influenza
Newcastle disease

Of lesser importance are the LIST B diseases. Their definition runs as follows:

"Transmissible diseases which are considered to be of socio-economic and/or public health importance within countries and which are significant in the international trade of animals and animal products."

This group includes such diseases as: Rabies, Heartwater, Tuberculosis, New and Old World Screw worm, Brucellosis, and many others.

Recent events such as the BSE epidemic in Europe and the outbreaks of Nipah virus in Malaysia shown that even "unclassified" diseases can have severe economic or trading implications, especially when there is a link to public health.

FAO/EMPRES: a new emphasis

On taking office in January 1994, the new Director-General of FAO decided that the Organisation should be better focused in championing the goal of enhanced world food security and the fight against transboundary animal diseases and plant pests as outbreaks of such diseases or pests can result in food shortages, destabilise markets and trigger trade measures. A new programme with two sub-components was established: one to combat plant pests and diseases, and one to fight livestock diseases. These programmemes fell under the umbrella of EMPRES - Emergency Prevention Systems for transboundary diseases of animals and diseases and pests of plants.

This put livestock diseases something of a different light: transboundary diseases were now a specific target, and they are defined thus:

"Those diseases that are of significant economic, trade and/or food security importance for a considerable number of countries; which can easily spread to other countries and reach epidemic proportions; and where control/management, including exclusion, requires co-operation between several countries."

EMPRES has classified transboundary animal diseases into three flexible categories. These are:

•Epidemic diseases of **strategic importance**, namely rinderpest, foot-and-mouth disease and contagious bovine pleuropneumonia (CBPP) - these are accorded top priority by EMPRES at the global level. However, regions or countries can have a country-/region-specific set of strategic diseases, as well.

•Diseases requiring ***tactical attention*** at the international/regional level, e.g. Rift valley fever, lumpy skin disease, Peste des Petits Ruminants (PPR), Newcastle disease, African swine fever (ASF) and classical swine fever

•***Emerging*** or ***evolving*** diseases, e.g. BSE, porcine reproductive and respiratory syndrome (PRRS)

The diseases in the first two groups - diseases of strategic and tactical significance - have a particular danger in that their occurrence can evolve into epidemics which may threaten populations in a region, and have dire potential consequences in terms of international trade. When is a disease occurrence an epidemic? This is notoriously difficult to define. One definition given is "*The occurrence in a community or region of cases of an illness, specific health-related behaviour, or other health-related events clearly in excess of normal expectancy.*" (J.M. Last)

Where a disease is unknown in an area or has been absent for a long time, only one or two cases may qualify as an epidemic and warrant immediate attention. Where a disease has been present at a fairly constant prevalence level for some time, a marked upswing in the number of cases seen may signal a change in status from endemic to epidemic and will require investigation.

Thus the primary role of surveillance is to detect these changes in status early enough to take action. It means having the ability to detect a new incursion, or changes in present status, and presents a challenge to veterinary services in countries around the world. Renewed attention is being given to Transboundary Animal Diseases (TADs), many of which have their greatest impact in those very countries where surveillance (for many reasons) may be weakest.

Early Detection

The key to success in handling animal disease epidemics is early detection. If a disease can be detected very early in the phase of epidemic development, the possibility exists that it can be arrested and eliminated before it actually inflicts damage. Early detection presupposes that there is a surveillance system in place that will bring infection to light when it is first seen. The country's veterinary authorities are then placed in the position of being able to manage the problem before it becomes uncontrollable, thus protecting the local livestock industry and ensuring food security for those closely dependent upon livestock.

That is why this manual is all about surveillance. Early detection enables early warning and an early reaction. Surveillance is the primary key to effective disease management.

For more information on early reaction, the reader is referred to the FAO publication, "*Manual on the preparation of national animal disease emergency preparedness plans.*"

The need for surveillance

Surveillance has as its main purpose, early detection of disease. The sooner a disease is found before it makes progress along the epidemic curve, the better. The developing world is full of examples of countries with devastated livestock agriculture and severe economic losses incurred as a result of having found out too late. When the perceived threat of livestock epidemics recedes into the background, and there are spending cuts to be made, official Veterinary Services are usually the first to suffer, with a concomitant loss of ability to detect disease.

Thankfully, there are also examples of countries that did detect the very first outbreaks of disease, and were able to mobilise forces to neutralise them before they spread. It is much easier to tackle a disease problem in a small corner of a country where it is only necessary to deal with a small animal population, than to get to grips with a developing epidemic that is spreading on many fronts.

So much for surveillance and early detection. Surveillance has other roles, as well. One of these is monitoring the spread of a disease in order to manage it effectively. Knowing how fast a disease is spreading, in which directions it is going and the size of the populations threatened are all key factors in resource mobilisation. One needs to know how much vaccine to purchase, how many staff to deploy and where they should be deployed, the length of the cold chain that will be involved, and so on. Even when a disease is not present, but is the subject of regular vaccination campaigns (as in buffer zones), good surveillance will give a good idea of where to vaccinate and how many doses of vaccine to take along.

Surveillance plays an important role in the monitoring of progress in control and eradication programmemes. It is important to have in idea of whether the programme is successful (in other words, whether disease incidence is being reduced) in order to assess the efficacy of the control mechanisms being used. In this sense, surveillance becomes even more crucial during the eradication phases of the OIE pathways for various diseases. In these phases, it becomes necessary to prove the absence of a disease rather than to detect its presence: here, carefully planned surveillance actions are of the utmost importance.

What is surveillance?

The word "surveillance" has been used by epidemiologists for some considerable length of time, often interchangeably with "monitoring", and it is only recently that serious thought has been given to defining the two words.

Surveillance may be thought of as having a broad definition, in the sense of watching a population closely in order to see if a disease makes an incursion. The object of surveillance is early detection of disease. For the purposes of this manual, a **definition of surveillance** could then be given as:

"All regular activities aimed at ascertaining the health status of a given population with the aim of early detection and control of animal diseases of importance to national economies, food security and trade."

Monitoring, on the other hand is a more specific activity/ies that will follow as part of an early reaction should surveillance activities indicate introduction of disease. It will focus more specifically on the identified disease in order to ascertain changes in prevalence level, rate and direction of spread. **Monitoring** can thus be **defined** as:

"All activities aimed at detecting changes in the epidemiological parameters of a specified disease."

It should be pointed out that many of the techniques used to implement monitoring can be used in surveillance, and vice versa - and in fact, in practice, the distinction between the two often becomes blurred. As this is a practical book, the blurring will be noticeable in the text that follows. Readers will find much that is value in these pages, no matter whether they are anxiously waiting for a disease that they hope will never appear, or nervously following the progress of a disease they wish hadn't broken out. The distinction is more in the objectives than in the techniques applied.

Surveillance efforts, although as all-encompassing as possible are by their nature, are often not planned to be aiming at a particular confidence level in their execution, whereas monitoring is usually mathematically planned and aims to follow disease dynamics with a certain measure of precision. Readers should be aware that doors are open for bias and error in both monitoring and surveillance, and should consult reputable textbooks on epidemiology to ascertain sources of error and bias, and how these are best counteracted. Mention will be made of many of the pitfalls of the different activities in the text. As mentioned earlier, this is a practical "how to" manual on information gathering and management, and the reader will want to make use of other texts for a fuller background on many of the concepts introduced here.

Surveillance on the ground

Surveillance Planning
Although perhaps not always mathematically precise, disease surveillance is not a haphazard action, but a meticulously planned and managed activity. It involves the deployment of personnel who will be moving in the field in a carefully programmed manner, using various methodologies to detect signs of livestock disease. This manual assumes that since the control of disease epidemics is in the greater public interest, it will be official veterinary staff who are involved in doing the work of surveillance for those diseases. Obviously, not all governments will have large armies of veterinary personnel; staffing levels will vary according to budgetary constraints and the importance of the livestock industry; this manual endeavours to deal with such differences.

Putting a surveillance system in place

National governments must realise that animal disease surveillance is a key function of their national veterinary services. Once that is an accepted principle, there is a need to agree on the **need** for a properly structured and administered system. Having a properly implemented and utilised system will require co-operation from a number of stakeholders - the official veterinary service (management and field staff), other extension staff, private veterinarians, farmers and other organisations that might be operating on the ground, for example NGOs. Assuming at this point that it is the official veterinary service that is initiating the drive, it will have to make contact with these stakeholders, explain the intention, and enlist their support. It will also require transparency, as those who are involved in data supply and collection will want to see that the information they supply is actually put to use.

In developing countries, properly supervised sub-professional groups (veterinary assistants, auxiliaries and community animal health workers and the like) are often important elements in surveillance systems, and must be singled out for special training.

The next item on the agenda would be to agree on the **objectives** of such a system. A specimen set of objectives might be:

- the early detection of livestock diseases of economic/food security/public health importance
- enabling early reaction to such diseases
- correct identification of resource needs in the field so that existing resources can be correctly deployed in disease management
- provision of strategic decision-making support
- measurement of surveillance system performance

What would the **priorities** of such a system be? The first would be to identify the most important *diseases* in the country. Field staff (and farmers, for that matter) would need to be familiarised with these diseases, and at least know the basics about recognising them in order to be able to report their presence. There is obviously nothing wrong in reporting any disease through the system, no matter how insignificant it may seem; the problem comes in allocating resources for staff training - this is where decisions will have to be made about priority diseases. Time and training materials will have to be devoted to priority diseases.

Having identified priority diseases, the next step is to identify *priority areas*. It will probably also not be possible to direct resources equally throughout the country, and the areas where the identified diseases pose the greatest problem will have to be earmarked for the first resources in terms of training, staff, intensity of surveillance, etc.

It is likely that priorities will differ in different parts of a country, and that must be taken into account. While CBPP may be of importance in one province, trypanosomosis may be of greater importance in another. Planning of training and awareness creation will have to take such differences into account.

Beyond a country's borders, it may be that other diseases enjoy priority. In each region of the world, a different set of circumstances, with its own set of livestock diseases, exists. Being a responsible global citizen will require a country's veterinary service to be aware of regional priorities in terms if disease surveillance, and internal surveillance systems will also need to take account of these. Regional economic and political groupings often play a leading role in drawing up regional priority lists of animal diseases.

A final criterion in developing a priority list for surveillance is that of international disease reporting. Every country that is an OIE member will need to decide what OIE List A and B diseases are of local importance, how to detect these diseases, and how to report on them. Transboundary Diseases as defined by the FAO will also play a role in shaping surveillance systems. Defining priorities is therefore not purely a matter of local interest, but also a matter of sensitivity to international concerns. The greater the attention given to diseases that are transboundary in nature, the greater the opening for participation in international trade and economic advancement.

Targets must also be defined, as well as **responsibilities**. In the various priority areas, decisions will need to be made concerning staff deployment levels, and time-frames set. What will the frequency of surveillance inspections be in area? When will they start? If there is to be sero-surveillance, when will the first survey take place? Will there be regular serosurveys? Who will be responsible for each activity? Will computers be used? Do questionnaires need to be drawn up?

A proper management plan, defining priorities, targets, responsibilities, resource allocation and responsibilities must be drawn up and adhered to. The various elements that should be included in such a plan will be made clearer in the pages of this manual.

In drawing up a management plan, the normal information flow in a surveillance system will need to be taken into account, and every step in the flow properly monitored and controlled.

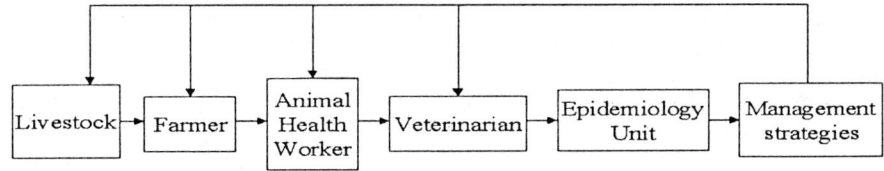

Information flow in Surveillance and

Livestock Disease Management

Surveillance for what?

If information is to be collected, it will have to be managed, and - most important - *used*. Data collection with no clear purpose is a waste of time and resources. One thing that data managers will have to define very clearly, is *what incident will trigger what action, and at what level*. The data that should be collected is that data which will lead to action.

For example, the first-time suspicion of a Transboundary Disease in an area will require immediate action by the local veterinarian - perhaps in terms of quarantine or movement control, and certainly in terms of follow-up. At management level, it may require further decisions in terms of publicity and redeployment of resources.

Exactly what action is taken by who, and under what circumstances, must be spelled out as a part of the surveillance system. It will obviously differ from country to country, and even from region to region within countries, and this type of planning rests firmly in the domestic arena. But it is planning that *must* be done.

Surveillance when and how?

It was mentioned earlier that surveillance is a planned activity, involving a carefully laid-out routine. The type and level of activity, the routine (frequency of activity in any area) are all determined by the country's veterinary management, in agreement with the various stakeholders, according to the criteria listed above.

Suffice it to say that whether government staff are combing an area in large numbers looking for a disease themselves, or whether a small team is conducting retrospective farmer interviews, the activity must be a planned activity that is worked into the annual activity plan.

A little extra time and resources spent on surveillance at the beginning will save a lot of time and money later on should a disease break out. Surveillance planning will include such things as deciding on how many staff members will be devoted to surveillance, the frequency of visits, distances to be travelled and transport requirements. Planning must be such that activities are evenly spread, not that one day is overburdened with work (creating the necessity for a "rush job") while another day's activities are very light. This kind of information is necessary not only for execution of the activity itself, but also for budgetary planning. For an example, see below:

Example of work programme

Month: June   **Week**: 1st week   **Name**: Tobias Malinga   **Duty station**: Kwela

Date	Village(s)	No. inspection points	Estimated km travel	Cost ($)
3	Kwela, Moshu	7	20	15.00
4	Elondo	9	18	13.50
5	Tsando, Ekoti	8	21	15.75
6	---------------------------------- Public Holiday --			

Having a fixed work plan means that the staff member knows exactly where he needs to be and when he needs to be there; and should supervisory staff need to monitor what he is doing, they know where to find him. Should the staff member need to be contacted in the field in an emergency, his whereabouts will be known. If the person is using a vehicle, the distance estimates in the work plan will also serve as a guide to indicate how closely the plan was adhered to.

Visits to the field must be planned in such a way that a single round trip will cover the biggest area possible. Surveillance teams (or individuals) should have areas demarcated for them, and should not overlap. Wherever possible, the same staff should be visiting the same areas every year – this enables the livestock owners to get to know the staff and build up trust in them, and enables the staff to get to know the area and the movements and habits of the people more intimately. Regular surveillance by the same staff member (preferably of the same ethnic group as the farmers being visited) builds mutual confidence and means that farmers will report diseases more readily.

Surveillance does not simply mean that a staff member "does the rounds" inspecting livestock or taking blood samples: it requires that the surveillance officer be involved in a constant process of informing and educating his farmers so that they will immediately recognise telltale disease signs and report their presence without delay. Extension activities could be incorporated into the surveillance plan, and certainly the official should be carrying a supply of information leaflets and/or posters giving details of diseases of local importance.

Surveillance: local needs vs national needs

The battle cry is usually to "keep surveillance focussed." Having a narrow focus for disease control activities will, however, often backfire. Diseases of importance to the national veterinary service are often not of importance at the grassroots level. Low profile rinderpest will almost certainly be of lesser importance to a rural community than concurrent endemic CBPP; ongoing surveillance for FMD in an area where the disease is normally absent (but perhaps occurs only every five or six years) will not gain a community's sympathy. Forcing an approach onto a community won't work, and will only cause resentment. Local communities need to feel that their needs are being catered for, and in order to gain co-operation, compromises will need to be made.

Shaping such compromises means listening to farmers, and taking other disease needs into account. It will certainly mean carrying out surveillance for a package of diseases rather than a single one. The logic for this concept is both economic and practical. The system put into place for surveillance of the critical target disease can easily capture data on other diseases in the same area. The sustainability of the system will be better secured as it will be viewed more positively at both the local and the national level. Furthermore, it should be remembered that even during a disease eradication process, there is a requirement for the surveillance system to demonstrate its capacity for those that are relevant for differential diagnosis.

Nevertheless within a broad-based national surveillance system, there will be a need from time to time for specific targeted surveillance programmes aimed at either specific and special awareness/early warning or in aid of special eradication programmes.

While targeting a broad range of diseases makes sense from the managemental and economic points of view, there is a lot to be said for surveillance "riding on the back" of a particular disease. Very often, it is a single disease (such as rinderpest or Foot-and-mouth disease) which causes a national scare and provides the impetus for putting a national surveillance network in place. Once resources are in place, moving from an emergency response to a proper surveillance system is only a very small step. Moving to wide-spectrum surveillance must ensure that impact scenarios can be constructed. Surveillance also means having the information necessary to predict what the consequences of other disease epidemics might be. Having secured the resources necessary to put a surveillance network in place, the same network must ensure its survival by justifying its economic importance on the national scene.

The same kind of reasoning applies to extension work. If surveillance personnel are equipped for extension (which they should be), then their extension materials should take account of local needs. Training must be provided on the recognition of a number of diseases, so that the network is "sensitive" to a varied repertoire of needs.

This is especially so where a network relies heavily on the reporting by farmers of disease outbreaks. If farmers feel confident about reporting diseases with which they are familiar, they will also feel easier about reporting occurrences that are foreign. The benefits work two ways: farmers feel that something is being done to assist them with their own identified needs, while the surveillance system will have a greater chance of detecting "exotic" diseases.

The flexibility to cope with ad-hoc needs

Much has been said above about having a planned surveillance schedule that runs for year after year. A routine programme is important, but it must not exclude *ad-hoc* needs. It should be possible to re-deploy staff to take care of new needs – for example, a need for heightened surveillance in a particular part of the country for a short while to guard against a threatening disease incursion. Reviewing surveillance programmes and their efficacy – and, if necessary, changing them to suit population shifts or disease patterns, is an important part of surveillance management.

Visual Surveillance

Having planned a surveillance programme, what types of surveillance could be undertaken? Probably the most popular – and one of the easiest and cheapest – is visual surveillance. Two kinds of visual surveillance can be distinguished: *direct* and *indirect*. For both types, the veterinary official visits all (or as closely as possible to all) farmers in the area allocated to him/her. This is less of a random sampling exercise and more of a census. It is carried out on a regular basis, any number of times per year, depending on staffing, budgetary constraints and the prevailing disease situation.

In *direct* visual surveillance, the observer physically inspects all animals and records what he sees in terms of disease. Probably the best way of doing this with cattle is to first observe them from a fairly close distance and run them slowly through a race/crush if one is available. Individual animals can be selected for closer examination should they appear unhealthy. Small ruminants are probably best looked at from as close a distance as possible in a pen. Again, those appearing sick can be singled out for closer examination. The official's findings are recorded on a pre-printed data questionnaire. It may be possible for the officer to take samples for laboratory confirmation, or even to perform a post-mortem, depending on his/her mobility and other logistics.

This approach assumes that the veterinary official involved – who is usually a lay person – has had fairly comprehensive training in recognising diseases of local importance, as well as diseases of national or international importance which might not occur locally on a regular basis.

With indirect surveillance, it is assumed that the livestock inspection frequency is very low, and therefore, while the official visits all possible livestock owners, he/she relies on their recall to gain details of diseases that affected their flocks and/or herds. While some may scoff at this kind of surveillance, it is important to note that most herders have an accurate knowledge of local diseases, and are usually fairly close to target when it comes to making diagnoses. If they aren't always all that accurate clinically (usually because there may be different diseases in an area with similar clinical pictures) there will be certain syndromes which usually have fairly descriptive names in the local vernacular. These names at least – and the approximate numbers of animals which were affected – can be recorded for further investigation if necessary. Usually, by closely questioning farmers about the clinical signs seen, it is also possible to arrive at a tentative diagnosis. Again, it is necessary for the veterinary staff to have a good idea of clinical signs and post mortem lesions to be able get all possible information out of the farmer.

It is important when questioning a farmer not to ask leading questions, or to use a questionnaire with "pre-cooked" clinical signs listed on it (if at all possible). Herders might be led to believe that this is a quiz where "yes" is the right answer, and may well report disease signs that were never seen.

In practice, of course, the two types of visual surveillance are never really separated. Usually, the veterinary staff member will inspect all the animals present, record what he sees, and then ask the farmer about all diseases that were seen since the previous inspection. All observations – both direct and indirect, are then recorded.

Sero-surveys
Sero-surveillance, while it may give a more "objective" view of the disease situation in an area (it measures antibodies rather than a lay person's conception of a disease), has its limitations. Among them are:

- Costs – of blood and serum tubes, needles, transport of samples to laboratories and the cost of testing.
- Lay staff will have to be trained in sample-taking.
- Suitable facilities (good crushes with working head-clamps) are not always available in rural areas.
- In some cultures, there may be strong objections to the taking of blood from live animals.
- Animals not always be handleable when it comes to taking samples.
- Because of the costs involved, the survey is more likely to be carried out on a small subset (a random sample) of population than on a larger cross-section of animals, and the question of sampling error then comes into play.
- The specificity (the probability that a non-diseased subject will be classified as diseased) and the sensitivity (likelihood that an exposed case will be classified as

exposed) vary from laboratory test to laboratory test for various diseases, and are never 100%. This also introduces inaccuracies into the surveillance effort.

Nevertheless, sero-surveillance is still more "objective" than visual surveillance, and for many diseases it can be used to get an idea of current prevalence and geographic distribution. The costs and other problems involved should not be a discouragement to use sero-surveillance. A well-planned random survey will carry benefits that should far outweigh its costs. In the case of rinderpest, sero-surveillance can be used for antigen detection (for investigating wild virus activity or proving absence of infection), while seromonitoring is used for post-vaccination antibody detection.

Planning a serological survey

First, the objective and the tests to be used must be clearly stated. If surveillance is for Rinderpest, what is being sought? Evidence of exposure to disease, or evidence of vaccination? Where? In what species? Is this part of an eradication process? If so, is it only going to be a zonal process or a national one? Once the objectives have been decided and the area/s to be surveyed have been delineated, other decisions have to be made.

What will the sampling units be? The primary sampling units will, in most cases, be herds. Herds, in developing countries, need definition, and these definitions will vary by geography, ethnic group and farming system. It might be a group of animals cared for by an individual, or it might be a group of animals owned by a collection of individuals. The secondary sampling units will then be individual animals. If the individual is important (eg. when trying to link clinical signs to antigen presence or an antibody titre), then identification of the individual becomes important - if not, one needs not be too concerned with secondary sampling units.

Once the type of sampling unit is known, and the survey area is defined, the next step is to draw up a sampling frame from which the psu's will be chosen. The sampling frame would be, for example, a list of all villages in the survey area, together with the livestock populations of each village.

The primary sampling units are then chosen by random sampling. Procedure for random sampling will not be discussed here (but a short summary is given in an appendix), as they are described in epidemiology textbooks, as well as FAO and OIE publications (eg. "Recommended surveillance procedures for disease and serological surveillance as part of the Global Rinderpest Eradication Programme (GREP)" IAEA/FAO, 1994). What is important is to determine the confidence limits (usually 95%) and the prevalence level which is desirable to detect beforehand, as this will, in turn, determine the size of the sample to be taken. How to calculate sample sizes is covered in many authoritative texts; it will not be given here.

Nomadic herds present a special problem. Very often, instead of doing a random village selection, one can do random selection of grid blocks from a map, enter the areas selected, and then sample a percentage of the animals found inside the block. This technique has been well described elsewhere.

Once the area to be covered, the size of the samples and the whereabouts of the herds to be sampled have all been worked out, the next (and more down-to-earth) stage of planning is reached. This will involve the following:

- Working out the needs in terms of how many teams will be sent into the field, how many vehicles are to be used, a sampling programme, and how many animals each team will have to bleed, how many members are required for each team. Sample tubes and accessories will have to be included as well as marker pens and ear tags (if identification of individual animals is important). Bear in mind extras such cool boxes and aids to animal handling. This will enable a budget to be drawn up for the entire exercise.

- Then comes the purchase of vacuum sampling tubes, needles and needle-holders, and any extras in terms of ropes, nose-tongs etc. Remember when purchasing vacuum tubes that provision will have to made for extra tubes in case of breakages and defective tubes. It is important to bear in mind that serum sampling requires an extra set of tubes for decanting serum from blood (this is often done in the field), and that the total number of tubes required is thus double the number of samples to be taken.

- Tubes must then be marked. If individual animals are important (e.g. in Rinderpest follow-up) a marking code will have to be developed for the village/settlement and the individual. If the individual animal is not important (e.g. in a CBPP sampling exercise where serology is of value in identifying infected herds only), then the village code is of importance on the tubes. This code will have to be used on the blood tube, the serum tube and the sample form. All of this is best done in advance.

- Each team will have to be fully briefed on the programme to be followed, and issued with all items of equipment needed. Small things like pens, sample record forms/questionnaires, clipboards, extra marker pens for sample tubes, etc should not be forgotten. The individual villages or farms must be clearly identified to the teams, as well as the numbers of animals to be bled at each place. Arrangements must be made for transport and cooling of sample tubes - cool boxes should be provided for.

- If teams are going to be in the field for a number of days, they will need to camp out. Blood samples can be allowed to settle overnight, and the serum decanted early the next morning - alternatively small hand centrifuges (fairly impractical for large numbers of samples) can be used to separate the serum. When sampling teams are spending time in the field, other needs, such as food, camping equipment, extra petrol and essential motor spares must be remembered.

Something often forgotten by field staff planners of serosurveys is to make all necessary arrangements with the laboratory analysing the samples. The laboratory should have the technical ability to perform the tests required, and should be informed of the arrival of the samples well in advance in case extra resources need to be reserved for the job.

"Passive" surveillance

Most ordinary surveillance routinely carried out falls into the category of passive surveillance. In this case, there are routine programmes that run - usually partly directly visual, or indirect, relying on farmer interviews and notification - basically to survey the landscape for livestock diseases and to detect and changes in status. This is probably the most important, and is a key element in early warning. The word "passive" should be seen as a characterisation of technique and not a sign of lowered importance of the work done.

"Active" surveillance

Much has been made of the concepts of "passive" and "active" surveillance. Passive surveillance is usually thought of as regular - and perhaps infrequent - visits to an area by veterinary staff to assess the local animal situation and determine livestock populations. It would include voluntary disease reporting by farmers, traders and perhaps other individuals such as private veterinarians.

"Active" surveillance entails frequent and intensive efforts to establish the presence of disease in an area. Examples:

- A disease threatens from just across a country's border. The threatened country will mount frequent livestock inspections, perhaps coupled with specific clinical observations ("mouthing" for FMD, close examination of mucosae for lesions and discharges for rinderpest). As an adjunct to this, serum samples might also be taken frequently.
- Frequent patrolling of borders or *cordons sanitaire* to detect and follow up illegal livestock movements.
- When a disease is suspected in an area, active surveillance techniques are often used to confirm its presence - or, hopefully, its absence.
- Active surveillance is of great importance in supporting official declarations to eradicate disease. Once the declaration has been made, it is up to country concerned to meet all requirements for proving freedom from disease, and finally, freedom from infection (eg. rinderpest, CBPP).
- Countries may be required, as part of livestock trade protocols, to prove absence of a certain disease (eg. Foot-and-mouth disease, Tuberculosis, BSE).

Any activity which is frequent, intensive and aims at establishing the presence or absence of a specific disease, could be described as "active" surveillance.

Once the presence of a disease is confirmed, and similar techniques are then used to follow trends in its development, this would (at least in terms of current terminology) be called "monitoring".

There is no doubt that active surveillance activities can be expensive and time-consuming. There are benefits, however, that in the long run will outweigh the costs. In the first instance, beginning active surveillance (at least for diseases such as rinderpest and CBPP) means that vaccination has ceased, and huge amounts spent on blanket vaccination campaigns will be saved. Secondly, there are trade benefits to be gained - eventual proof of disease absence will allow the opening-up of hitherto untapped markets.

Abattoirs and slaughter slabs

These are a valuable source of data, particularly when it comes to diseases which present laboratory diagnostic difficulties, such as CBPP. It has rightly been said that abattoirs are "the post mortem halls of the nation" and are a goldmine of information. Export abattoirs are always closely monitored by veterinary officials, and instituting a reporting system to extract information from them would present no problem. Smaller abattoirs and slaughter-slabs present something of a problem in that there may not be enough official staff to keep them under surveillance. Possible solutions to this would include the following:

- Entering into agreement with those running smaller facilities - or even butchers at slaughter slabs - to alert the authorities in the event of a possible transboundary disease being detected on slaughter. This will require some investment in terms of basic meat inspection training and the recognition of characteristic lesions, but it may be well worth the outlay.
- Random inspection of slaughter slabs or small abattoirs by officials who might spend a day or half a day keeping watch on the proceedings at a particular place, and then move to other duties - or to the next slaughter slab.
- Intensive inspection activities could be reserved only for those facilities perceived as being in "high risk" areas.

The kinds of information required here would be such things as species, origin of animals slaughtered, lesions seen, condition suspected. During the eradication phases of a disease pathway, surveillance would have to be organised such that:

* it was random
* it covered the required number of animals at a 95% confidence level to give reasonable assurance of the absence of disease.

Rapid appraisals

Rapid Appraisals go by many names (Rapid Rural Appraisal, Participatory Rural Appraisal, Particpatory Epidemiology, Sondeo Method, etc). The basic idea of the Rapid Appraisal is collect information in data-sparse areas, places that are marginalised, remote, inhabited by nomads, inhospitable, infrastructure-poor - whatever adjectives one might choose for neglected areas, whatever the reason for the neglect might be.

Rapid Appraisals provide a means for data collection which would otherwise not be there: the data may be limited in scope, inaccurate or biased - but it *is* data, in certain vast areas of the developing world where information is virtually non-existent, any data are better than none. Such data may not be statistically valid, but will at least provide an indication of what is happening "out there" - and where it is happening. It is based on rural livestock owners' impressions, but their impressions are often very accurate.

Many possible "tools" are available for appraisal work, but the end result is usually an unstructured/semi-structured interview during which the interviewer tries to capture some form of data, at least in a semi-structured form. The essential ingredients are (a) to know exactly what information is required, (b) how to capture it fairly informally, and (c) how to structure it so that it can finally be computerised (if necessary) and analysed.

In summary, Rapid Appraisals make use of the following tools to gather information:

- Background studies of historical, demographic, epidemiologic and geographic information to become acquainted with the area under study (including previous consultants' reports, scientific papers, population census data, official reports and maps).
- Interviews with "key informants" - community leaders, church leaders, government officials, health workers, veterinarians, NGO workers and others in contact with the local people who can provide information on what is happening in an area.
- Group interviews with farmers (need careful organising and chairmanship to ensure fair representation of poor and elite, and to ensure that individuals do not dominate the group).
- Gender analysis - using men to talk to men - to find out what they do, when they do it, and what they know - particularly with reference to livestock diseases. Similarly, women must be used to interview women. This type of technique may not always be acceptable in some communities, but when it is, it should be exploited to the full. Women usually work more with poultry and small livestock, and their knowledge of diseases in this field is extensive and invaluable.
- Direct observation - often, spending a day watching how people in rural areas handle their farming system provides essential information that will give a better understanding of livestock management, and how to handle disease problems. Linkages within the farming system (crop-livestock) may also be better understood. Walking around a farming area will provide valuable impressions of livestock, husbandry methods and the status of the ecology.
- A very good means of carrying out appraisals is the use of community animal health workers or "veterinary scouts". Such people provide a basic service to the community in their private capacity and are remunerated by the community for services rendered (usually medical treatments, or simple procedures such as castrations). Because of their more specialised knowledge, they are excellent sources of information for appraisals. Of course, such people need training and initial drug and equipment supplies at the outset, and this will cost money. Such schemes also do not always work, but in communities where they are self-sustaining, costs are limited to an initial outlay only.

When using appraisal techniques to gather disease data, one must bear in mind the various sources of error and bias:

- Farmer recall. The longer the period between visits to an area, the longer is the recall period required from farmers. This may lead to all sorts of errors in observation, and a group interview - where farmers get the opportunity to validate each others' observations - may be helpful in this regard. Interviews with other informants may also provide a means of cross-checking information, but care must be taken to ensure that informants are really in contact with what is happening at grassroots level, and that their inputs are credible.
- Interviewer bias. Interviewers may have their friends among the more influential farmers and tend towards interviewing them at the expense of poorer farmers. In addition, interviewers might have their own ideas about what is important and may tend to miss the "smaller" details that often make the difference.
- Travel limitations. Restricted ability to travel due to poor roads and inhospitable countryside may miss the more remote areas where any number of disease problems

may be brewing. This may also be a stumbling-block to follow up: even if a possible transboundary disease is identified in an isolated area, there may be a reluctance to follow it up and confirm the rumour due to the distance and difficulty of access.

- Community desires for service provision. Farmers may be tempted to exaggerate their disease problems in the hope that this will attract more services from the government.
- Information may "get lost" between interviewer and interviewee if interpreters have to be used.

Despite the fact that Rapid Appraisals are fraught with problems that amount to a statistician's nightmare, they are essential in areas where staff are thin on the ground and frequent and intensive surveillance is not possible. They provide useful information on the *disease situation* in the area, the *farming systems*, the *distribution of people and livestock*, and on *trading routes* - where they run, how and when they are used. Trading routes are notoriously difficult to document, and Rapid Appraisal tools provide a means of recording these routes (which need updating from time to time).

Another important use of Appraisals relates to the provision of baseline *economic data* for the calculation of losses due to disease impact. A number of appraisals, using interviews combined with direct observation in an area, will give an idea of livestock production. Cash values can later be imputed to these estimated production parameters in order to calculate the economic cost of a disease epidemic should it strike the area.

The role of Laboratories in surveillance programmes

A final word here about the role of laboratories in veterinary surveillance. Diagnoses (or tentative diagnoses) can be made in many ways:

- Visual (by non-professional field staff)
- Clinical observation (by veterinarians)
- Post-Mortem evaluations (usually by veterinarians)
- Simple laboratory examinations (blood smears, faecal examinations, impression smears)
- Laboratory methods (serology, tissue culture, bacteriology, histopathology, etc)

Often, laboratories are thought of as having relevance only in serological surveys. However, it is imperative that laboratory backup be obtained for as many diagnoses as possible. It is essential in cases where an epidemic disease is suspected for the first time in an area that samples be taken for confirmation of the diagnosis. Where the diagnosis is uncertain, repeated follow-ups, with laboratory sampling, must be made in an effort to either confirm or exclude the disease. Where it is known that a certain disease has become endemic, confirmation of each individual focus becomes unnecessary, but 10-20% of cases must always be confirmed to ensure that the epidemiological picture has not changed and that another disease, different in epidemiology but similar in appearance, has entered.

For these reasons, the presence of a strong laboratory diagnostic service, subservient to the official veterinary service, and answerable to it, is absolutely essential. Laboratory services are an essential backup to what is being done by field service staff.

It is also necessary - and this is often forgotten - that field staff (including veterinarians) be regularly briefed on the kind of samples needed for the various diseases threatening in an area, and that they are also familiar with the requirements for preserving, packaging and transporting such samples.

Maintaining laboratory norms

Laboratory testing needs standardisation so that, for example, the results of serosurveys analysed by different labs are comparable. This means that laboratories need to belong to networks where the same reagents and methods are used in the same test; where experience and expertise is shared; and where use is made of reference laboratories. A chain of OIE and FAO reference laboratories has been established for this purpose. The FAO/IAEA Joint Division has also been established to assist with standardisation of tests, and for quality assurance. It is imperative that national veterinary laboratories make use of these services.

Surveillance in Resource-poor countries

Surveillance often presents itself as a thorny issue in developing countries because it is seen as a costly operation necessitating an enormous army of surveillance personnel on the ground. This need not be so, and judicious deployment of resources can often achieve what is needed without great expense.

Critical point identification

The first step in setting up a "low cost" surveillance system involves identifying *critical points* or *critical surveillance areas*. These would include:
- areas under direct threat of disease (perhaps due to the presence of a nearby focus)
- border crossings
- watering points or slaughter slabs near migration routes
- auction pens and other major livestock assembly points
- abattoir lairages

Resource deployment

The bulk of veterinary resources should then be deployed at these critical points, with high frequency surveillance designed to move staff amongst such points with relative rapidity for whatever type of surveillance is deemed appropriate - visual (for detecting clinical/pathological signs), detection of antibody, and detection of the causative agent. Such surveillance is fairly structured but not sufficiently randomised for movement along an OIE pathway. It would, however, qualify a country for entrance to a pathway if it gained sufficient evidence of clinical disease absence - the point is that the work would have to be restructured along more "scientific" lines in order to move further along an OIE pathway.

As an aside, it must be mentioned that strategic resource deployment may clash with equity goals - politicians may want to see a more "even" distribution of resources across the country. Careful explanation will have to be given for unequal resource deployment, with the assurance that once the disease problem is cleared up, personnel and equipment will once again be redistributed.

Surveillance frequency

The frequency of surveillance at these critical points is a matter of common sense and would have to be determined by the perceived risk of each point, with the higher risk points receiving the most frequent attention. Frequency of surveillance will, on the one hand, be determined by the frequency of population turnover (eg. along trade routes) and by the incubation period of the main disease feared at the time. In a relatively static livestock population at high risk to foot-and-mouth disease, for example, it would not make much sense for surveillance to be more frequent than fortnightly. On the other hand, financial constraints will also be a major determinant of frequency. Surveillance needs to be an intelligent trade-off between field realities and budgetary limitations.

Non-critical areas

All other parts of the country would be deemed to be *non-critical areas* where surveillance could consist of relatively infrequent visits by field personnel (perhaps once or twice per year) or annual Rapid Appraisals relying heavily on group interviews. Useful information can also be gathered from other existing networks - for example NGO workers, crop extension officers who may happen to be in the area, consultants, etc.

An essential item in any surveillance system is *farmer awareness*. Training local livestock owners in disease recognition and encouraging them to report the presence of any suspicious clinical signs is a very cost-effective means of improving the quality of disease surveillance, both in critical and non-critical areas. There may even be a possibility of a small incentive to be provided for evidence leading to the discovery of a disease - eg. a fee to be paid should a farmer submit part of a diseased lung for CBPP examination.

Data from private veterinarians is an important item not to be forgotten. Capture of this may be via questionnaires sent to them regularly; a legal requirement for them to report certain diseases to the authorities; and by making the use of an official government questionnaire obligatory when sending samples to the laboratory (in this way, data from laboratory submissions will enter the system automatically).

Ultimately, the exact type of surveillance adopted by a country is its own decision, based on disease risk and available resources. What is important is the issue of transparency. It is incumbent on each country to make the precise mechanics of its surveillance system known to neighbours and trading partners. This includes the identification of critical areas and non-critical areas, and the types of surveillance operational in each. Such transparency builds confidence, facilitates mutual risk analysis, and in the long run, will promote investment and trade.

Information Systems

Much will be said about information systems and information management in this manual - for a very simple reason:

once information has been gathered, something has to be done with it.

Three things must happen to information: firstly, it must be *managed*, controlled and quality-checked; secondly, it must be *analysed* in order to become more understandable, and thirdly, it must be *acted upon*. These three points will be emphasised repeatedly throughout this manual. For information to be an analysable and eventually useful for decision-making, it needs careful management and quality control.

What is an information system?

An Information System is the collection of data, people, procedures, hardware, software, files, and information required to accomplish an organised set of functions.

> *- Tom Adamson*

Basically, the constituents of an information system are:

People
- those who gather data
- those responsible for data input
- those responsible for data analysis

A storage/retrieval/analysis system - which in this day and age would usually consist of
- computer software
- appropriate computer hardware

A feedback delivery system
- mechanisms to ensure that processed data is fed back to data gatherers

An information system is nothing more than a large communication cycle, involving information transmission and reception. In any communication cycle, one person (the communicator) transmits information via a medium (the spoken word, the written word) to a recipient. In order to ensure that the concept transferred to the recipient's mind is what was originally in the communicator's understanding, and also to motivate the communicator's further participation in the interaction, there has to be feedback. During feedback, the recipient will communicate with the original transmitter of information in order to receive clarification, or to take action.

The diagram below illustrates the essential elements of the communication cycle.

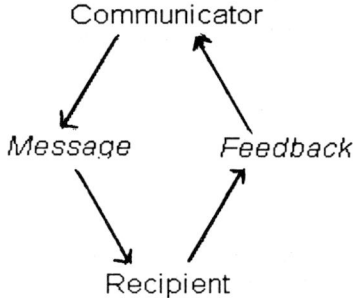

Elements of the Communication Cycle

A breakdown in any one of these elements will cause the breakdown of the entire cycle and communication will sooner or later come to a halt. This should be borne in mind when planning, and later when maintaining, the flow of information through a system. There needs to be a clearly defined flow of information with defined inputs, outputs and feedback. Suppliers of information need to know that the products of their labour are being put to good use, or their supply will dry up.

Structure and flow of veterinary information systems will be dealt with in greater detail later, suffice it to say at this stage that information is usually garnered from farmers by some kind of field worker, who will pass it up a chain to a central computer system, from where feedback will be transmitted back to the field.

Managing the system

Provision must be made for the position of system manager to run the system. Such a person will have to carry out the following functions:

- *Monitor data flow* into the system - and take follow-up action when flow slows down, or when inflow becomes abnormally large. Both could indicate abnormalities in the system which need to be remedied. A "drying-up" of data coming in could indicate a lack of motivation of field staff for a number of reasons (including poor feedback), or logistical problems among data gathering staff in the field. A "surge" of flow could mean that there is an upswing in disease incidence, or livestock population, or rampant data fabrication, or that the system had been functioning suboptimally before the surge, and it is now coming to an equilibrium.

- *Check data quality* - various parameters need checking. They vary from simple spellings to handwriting, looking for fabricated data, checking internal logic (for example, when a veterinarian reports zero deaths in an area, but in the same report describes post-mortem lesions). This might also mean cross-checking with data from other sources, providing direct feedback to suppliers of data and requesting them to verify what has already been submitted. The manager must be motivated enough - and have enough "clout" in the hierarchy - to take action when deficiencies come to light.

- Carrying out *data analysis* and ensuring that analysed information reaches decision-makers. This is an ongoing function, and disease data will need ongoing temporal and spatial analysis to look for trends in terms of increasing or decreasing incidence, spread of disease, etc. Vaccination data will need following-up to assess percentage coverage in vaccination campaigns. Again, the manager must not just be an observer. Disturbing trends demand remedial action, and no manager can afford to be a spectator.

- *Ensuring feedback* to the field. Field staff need to receive reports indicating the outcomes of trends in data, and what action is being taken to respond to these trends. This will encourage them to continue with their work, as they will see that what they do is constructive and helpful. It will also give them the opportunity to respond, and voice their opinions as to whether analyses made are reasonable, and whether actions taken are justifiable. In short, it gives them a stake in the system. At the same time, feedback needs to be given to livestock owners to encourage their further co-operation with field staff. This could take the form of information dissemination through pamphlets, posters or farmers' days. Once again, it effectively gives them a stake in the system, as well. It is the job of the information manager to ensure that such feedback is made, and that it reaches grassroot levels.

At country level, it is the *national epidemiologist* who is best placed to deal with overall information management. In large countries, some of his functions could be delegated to lower levels, but the overall responsibility for maintaining the integrity of the system should obviously - for simple reasons of accountability - be in the hands of one person.

Performance indicators – measuring efficacy of surveillance

Various parameters can be used to measure the efficacy of surveillance. These should be agreed upon during system formulation, and reviewed from time to time.

Such parameters should be monitored by the epidemiologist/information manager on a regular basis. Following trends every month is probably the best, and the epidemiologist should work out a simple monthly schedule to cater for routine activities such as data checking, reporting and analysis, and monitoring performance indicators. Examples of indicators that could be used are

* number of reports submitted/1000 head of livestock/district/month
* number of individual livestock inspections/staff member/month
* percentage of observed disease incidents for which laboratory samples were submitted
* percentage of suspected cases actually confirmed for any particular disease
* time lag from sample submission to final laboratory diagnosis

The Joint FAO/IAEA Division and EMPRES has proposed guidelines for use in Rinderpest surveillance for the GREP; these guidelines could be adapted to many situations. The information manager will need to establish the set of performance indicators best suited to his situation, and ensure that these are acted upon when the situation so demands.

Setting the goals; determining needs and outputs

To some extent, the outputs derived from an information system will determine what sort of inputs are required. In other words, when designing an information system, the first thing that must happen is that the system's future users must discuss their needs with a system designer. What sort of outputs are needed? To quote a trivial example, if we would like to know each month which diseases occurred, which species were affected, and how many animals were affected, it presupposes that the basic data will contain details such as the animal species affected, how many affected, the reporting date and the name of the disease suspected.

A good starting point would be to look at any existing manual system (often regular "monthly returns" that come to a supervisor and gather dust), and ascertain the inputs and outputs of that system. The new system in the process of conception might be able to build, at least to some extent, on what is already established. It will also show very clearly what kind of information is not used, and what could be improved upon to make it more useful.

Practicalities are important here. A natural tendency, while an information system is being designed, is to add all sorts of data requirements without any clear idea of whether they will be needed, and if they are ever needed, exactly how they will be used. Input requirements should be kept to an absolute minimum, remembering that the more complex the requirements, the greater the chances of error entering the system. The watchword is, "when in doubt, chuck it out".

For visual or clinical surveillance, for example, the following data items for each observed outbreak would be sufficient:

Locality*
Georeferences*
No. of cases*
No. of animals at risk
History and/or clinical signs
Tentative diagnosis*
Any treatment given
Any post-mortem lesions seen
Laboratory Results if available
Name of reporting officer
(Vet/Auxiliary etc)
Action taken

Date*
Species*
No. of deaths*
No. of animals examined
Clinical examination/field tests
Age category most affected
Sex category most affected
Any samples to a laboratory
Farming system
Category of reporting officer

* indicates minimum acceptable information

For sero-surveillance inputs (aggregation of these data at village/district level is satisfactory for a national database; information about each individual animal would be unnecessary) the following are reasonable guidelines:

Locality and date
Farming system

Species
Disease history of herd/flock

Vaccination history (past yr)	Age/sex category/ies bled
Vacutainer serial numbers	Disease being monitored
Test used	Sensitivity/specificity
No. positive	No. suspicious
No. negative	

Data requirements from abattoirs or slaughter slabs should include the following:

No. of animals in consignment (where applicable)	
Origin of animal/s (where known)	
Lesions seen	Condition diagnosed
Age most affected	Sex most affected
Samples sent to lab	Laboratory results if available
Category of reporting officer	

Being practical about data recording is important. The inputs required will determine the exact variables being recorded, and with increasing database complexity, management and analysis become increasingly difficult. This is particularly so where the database is a manual one - ie. not computerised, but it applies for computer-based systems as well. It will also influence the design and complexity of the questionnaire to be used. Again, the question will arise, what exactly is to happen to the variables being recorded? What will this information be used for? By whom? When? Is it really necessary?

"Information for the record" which will be used for analysis and as a basis for decision-making regarding disease control strategy must be distinguished from "information for immediate action" which will be communicated to the nearest veterinary officer for follow-up. For example, when recording data in a visual surveillance system, if disease was introduced into the area, there is little point in trying to use a computer database to record where the introduced animals came from, and what their destination was after they had infected animals already in the area. Apart from the fact that such information is notoriously difficult to computerise (and difficult to extract from a computer and even more difficult to use later), it is not that necessary for posterity. It is information that must be dealt with in a different way, as it obviously demands action in the form of following up the animal movement, finding the culprit animals and destroying or quarantining them - in other words, recent livestock movements must be reported to, and followed up by, the local veterinarian. This can then be dealt with in a narrative from the local veterinarian once he has finally dealt with the issue.

The matter of livestock movement in general is something that is tackled via a Rapid Appraisal rather than by a questionnaire specifically destined for a database, and which can be mapped rather than left to rot in a database.

Exactly how data are to be recorded and where is also an issue that needs decisions. Certain information may be necessary, but where and how is it to be recorded? Trying to put everything into a computer just because computers are fairly easy to come by, does not make sense, and such issues are a valid part of system creation.

A small aside is perhaps necessary at this point. While potential stakeholders in a computer system may be well-meaning, and have very genuine information needs, care must be taken to ensure that the system remains simple, with a direct information flow, a manageable number of inputs, and simple, clear outputs. The system designer must take a strong lead in the initial planning and be prepared to veto ideas that may detract from the efficiency of the system. The old adage about "the camel being a horse that was designed by a committee" can certainly be true when applied to information systems that are designed to accommodate too many "needs"!

Detail has been given above as to what sort of variables should be recorded. In large hierachical information systems, it should be remembered that such detail is probably only necessary at the lowest level of input and analysis. In a very large country, with a livestock population of many millions, it is unlikely that the national epidemiologist will need to know the exact clinical signs observed in a specific village, or the name of the diseased animals' owner. In a similar vein, when international disease reporting is undertaken to regional or global bodies, this kind of detail is also unnecessary. At higher levels of a system, basic information needs will be limited to such variables as the locality where the observation was made, the numbers and species of animals affected, the diagnosis made, and whether and how it was confirmed. These considerations must be borne in mind where large systems are planned.

What is important at national level, is that animal disease data not be "buried" and forgotten in common national records, but be passed to national epidemiologists for early analysis and further action, even if action has already been taken in the field. Such data must be readily accessible to veterinary management. Data should always be looked at when "fresh"!

Computerisation

As mentioned above, computers have become smaller, cheaper, user-friendly, more readily available and more robust. They can be taken into all sorts of environments and programmes are available that will perform a great variety of functions. But just as horses are more suited to certain terrain than the motor car, so we must remember that computers, for all of their hi-tech functionality, simply can't do everything. Computerisation, put bluntly, is not a panacea.

What it will do, what it won't do

Computers will not replace good personnel. They do not reach far-off stock owners and collect data. Trite though it may seem, having a computer doth not a system make. The system design must, first and foremost, incorporate people and their abilities, and make provision for extensive training in the use, completion and submission of data questionnaires. In the ordinary course of events, input questionnaires should never be completed by farmers and by those unschooled in their use; only by properly trained personnel. The first principle of data recording is, and always will be, "garbage in - garbage out".

Computers will not check data for you. They will not detect fabricated data, problems with data logic, nor will they improve poor handwriting on data forms. Such work must be done at field level by the most senior staff member available before forms are dispatched to the computer centre for typing-in.

Computers cannot replace the epidemiologist. Computers are simply data storage and retrieval devices. They cannot make judgements on data quality, notice disease trends, contact field veterinarians to ascertain their feelings on the current disease situation, or recommend a course of action. While the foregoing may seem glaringly obvious, it is all too often forgotten by those who want to create the "perfect system" without realising the crippling limitations of computer technology.

Computers are not a short-cut to easy data storage for all types of variables, either. They can be used for storing relatively simple numeric and non-numeric variables, and should only be used for this purpose. The examples given above of computerising livestock movements and storing trade routes are very fitting in the veterinary context. Another "variable" that must not be overlooked is a very simple one - the "gut feeling" of the field veterinarian. The field vet is in touch with farmers and field staff, he knows the conditions of the pasture, the livestock and the local market; he understands the way diseases behave in his area where he may have worked for some years. To computerise this? Impossible - which is why regular personal communication with headquarters is always important.

Computers also do not write interesting reports and do imaginative analyses, nor do they give constant encouragement to field staff. They may store data, but making sense of what is stored is, in the end, a human function. To calculate is computing, to interpret is human.

The centrepiece of any information system is not the computer, or the programmes installed on it: it is the people who run the system, and most particularly the epidemiologist who stands at the centre and directs operations. Without a dedicated, enthusiastic and "wide-awake" epidemiologist, the system will crash as surely as it will when the computer suffers a power failure.

National Computer systems

There is often a tendency to try to over-computerise, which can be fatal. In other words, some would have a computer in every district veterinary office - after all, what could be easier than local data input and simple electronic transfer to the central database. This concept has several major shortcomings:

- Who will be responsible for data input? And who will check it before it is transmitted upwards to the central computer? A busy veterinarian will certainly not type in large numbers of data forms reaching his office, and it will be left to a clerk. What of the work load already carried by the clerk? Or will one need to employ an army of data input clerks to cope with each district office? Data input is a very monotonous but highly demanding job that requires high standards of accuracy. Ordinary office clerks are usually unable to cope with such work, and when it is imposed on them, the results are often disastrous - slapdash and shoddy, with a wide variation in data quality between various staff members. In addition, if good data entry clerks are employed, their capabilities are usually such that they could easily cope with work from a number of districts simultaneously.

- Who will maintain the system? A huge network of computers strung out across the countryside means regular breakdowns, staff having problems with software, power failures, etc. This implies a number of technicians to keep order, and ensure a smooth flow of information.

- More importantly, who will pay? The more computers, the more connections, the greater the cost - the cost of maintaining the large number of machines, regular upgrades, and paying for the connectivity which will, obviously, be supplied by the national 'phone company.

Large numbers of staff with sophisticated, sprawling computer networks certainly have their place in developed countries, but in developing countries the secret is rather to start too small than too big. If one takes a convenient number of 20 to 25 veterinary districts to one computer, then it is quite practical to say that in large countries, a small computer unit at regional/provincial level could handle the inputs from those administrative divisions and than pass the data on to the central unit. In very small countries, a single central data input and processing unit would be sufficient. Admittedly, one would have to trust to national postal system to get data questionnaires to the input unit, but that is often preferable to trusting a strung-out computer network with all of its associated complications. The easiest way to handle this would be for each station to post all of its inputs on a regular basis (fortnightly; monthly) to its computer unit, and to keep duplicates (carbon copies are cheapest) of all questionnaires in reserve.

Managing the flow

When designing an information system, it is important to construct a flow diagram of how data flow in the system is envisaged, and what the various control points will be. This will of great importance in managing the system once it is running.

In general, the flow of data in the case of visual surveillance will be:

Farmer → Animal Health Worker → Veterinarian → Epidemiology Unit → Analysis & Feedback → Management Decisions

In the case of sero-surveillance, it will be slightly different:

Farmer/animals → Samples & Info → Laboratory → Results → Epidemiology Unit → Analysis & Feedback → Management Decisions

Having determined the route of flow, the next important step is to determine exactly what will happen at each step. Sending data straight from the field to the Epidemiology Unit, and then typing it directly into a computerised database would be foolhardy. Checking and validation mechanisms must be built in along the path to the database.

Taking the case of visual surveillance as an example, a more detailed flow diagram would look like this:

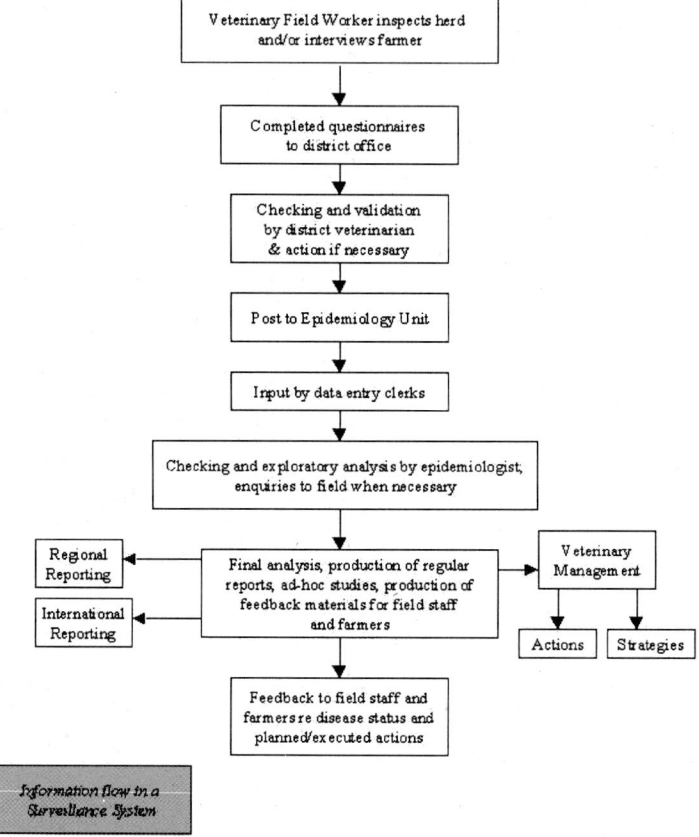

There are a number of "lines of defence" in data protection. The first is the person actually collecting the data. Such people should have clear handwriting, an ability to work with people and extract information from them, and a reputation for honesty.

They should be clearly briefed on what they are doing and why they are doing it. The importance of their work must be emphasised. Obviously, if the person collecting the information is a veterinarian, the foregoing points should not be a problem, however, in many cases the data collection staff will be community animal health workers or veterinary assistants, or similar groups.

The next line of defence is the veterinary district office. Here the form must be carefully checked by the district veterinarian. He is the one most familiar with the district situation, and is closest to the ground. This is the last opportunity to, if necessary, go back to the field and re-check the information before it is transferred to the epidemiology unit. **It is also the first opportunity for action**. If any suspicion of a transboundary disease is detected and reported, the district veterinarian must act immediately. There is no point in waiting for the data to be analysed by the national epidemiologist before doing anything about a disease outbreak.

Items to be checked by the district veterinarian would include:

- Legibility of writing on the questionnaire form. Ensuring readability at this level saves expensive phone calls from data input clerks later on.

- Correctness of spelling, particularly of place names. If geographic co-ordinates of places are included, these must also be checked.

- Internal logic. If a diagnosis of disease is made, but, for example, zero animals are reported as affected, the field worker has made an error which needs correction.

- Information must be realistic. If 100 animals are reported sick in an area where herd sizes average only 40, the farmer has probably exaggerated his problem to the field worker - or the field worker has not visited the farmer and has deliberately fabricated the data.

- Data encoding. If on-form encoding is used (see later), the codes used must be checked for correctness.

Only once the district veterinarian is completely satisfied that everything possible has been done to check and verify the data, should he submit the forms for computerisation.

The next line of defence is the data input clerk. They will obviously complain about poor handwriting, but experienced clerks will often detect other anomalies, such as incorrect place names, the diagnosis of a disease in an area where that particular disease does not normally occur, and so on.

The most important "data sifter" is, of course, the epidemiologist. His job will involve preliminary analyses to see what is in the database, follow-up communications to field veterinarians, and the detection of fabricated data. Additionally, he will be on the lookout for trends in disease spread, and for unusual occurrences that will alert him to possible problems brewing in the field.

The epidemiologist will be watching performance indicators, not only as far as field staff are concerned, but also checking the work of input clerks to determine typing errors. Errors can be quantified, for example as x errors per 100 questionnaires. Very often, the easiest way to look for input errors is to get input clerks to check each others' work. Although this will reduce the epidemiologist's work load, it will not free him from the need to carry out spot checks.

Complex systems

Ideally, there are a number of data sources that should be tapped. Although the means of collection of information, as well as storage format, will obviously differ, the streams of data will all flow into the same management system, to be analysed under the auspices of the one person, and to inform the decisions of the same veterinary service. Data may come from the field (veterinarians, lay staff), from abattoirs, and via laboratories (serosurveys, confirmatory sampling). This makes the flow more complex, and data checkpoints will increase in number, but the principles described above will remain the same.

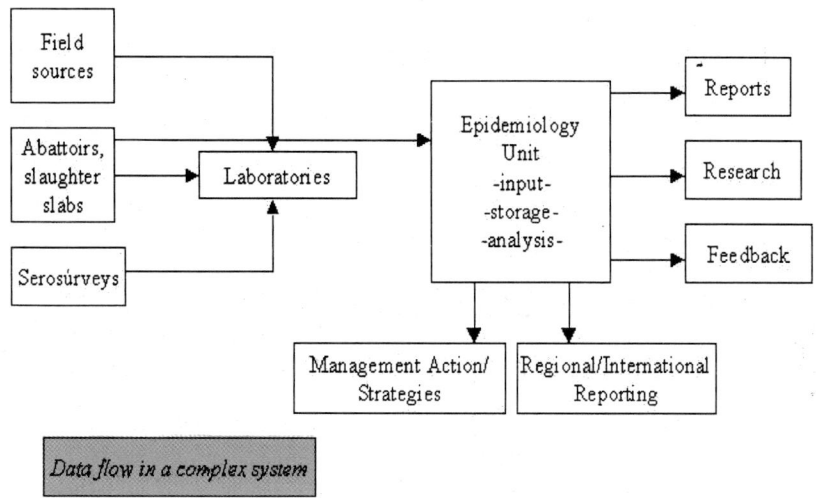

Data flow in a complex system

Information backup

Any information system must have a data backup capacity. Backups are kept in a variety of ways:

- duplicate copies of completed questionnaires at field offices.

- original copies of completed questionnaires, sorted according to district and month at the data input centre.

- electronic backups of data that has been stored on computer. Data may be backed up on tapes, diskettes, or compact disk, but _it must be backed up_. Some computer systems make provision for automatic daily backups, and these can be timed to take place after hours. In the absence of an automatic backup facility, data should be backed up at least once a week, so that if a computer crash occurs, the amount of information that has to be re-entered is minimised.

When making backups, especially onto tapes or CDs, the "grandfather-father-son" principle should be followed. If, for instance, the first backup is made on CD no. 1, the next on CD no.2 and the third on CD no. 3, then to make the fourth backup, the user will revert to CD no. 1. This ensures that the most recent backup is still available and unscathed should a crash actually occur during the backup process.

Running a system without a computer

It may seem unusual to include this topic in a manual written in the computer age, but the fact is that information systems can exist without computers, and in some cases, they simply have to. In far-flung areas where electricity supply is erratic or non-existent, in very poor countries or regions, or in small projects run by NGOs, computers may be inappropriate, impractical or simply too expensive.

In such cases, data are stored on large tables called tabulation sheets. Each column in the sheet will contain one of the variables to be recorded, while each row of the table will represent the information contained on a single questionnaire. It is self-evident that questionnaires will have to be short and simple, and data volumes low! Data entry staff will transfer data from the completed questionnaires to the tabulation sheet by hand.

An example of a tabulation sheet is given below:

Month	Place	Disease	Species	# Sick	# Dead	Signs	Officer
April	Kaluga	RP	Bov	3	6	diarrhoea	Ncube, B
April	Bukali	RP	Bov	1	10	diarrhoea	Ncube, B
April	Songa	CBPP	Bov	5	2	coughing	Ncube, B
April	Ongashi	Rabies	Cap	0	1	aggressive	Golan, J

On a monthly basis, data can be analysed using a tally sheet, for example:

Month:	April			
Diseases: (sick + dead)	Rinderpest	CBPP	LSD	Rabies
	3+6 = 9 1+10 = 11	5+2 = 7	0	1
Totals:	20	7	0	1

Such analyses can be done (as in the above example) per disease, or per village, per species - whatever the need might dictate, but they must be done by hand, and the database must be small enough to make allowance for such work.

More will be said about computerising data later.

Questionnaire design

Questionnaires can be used in a number of ways. Firstly, they can be used as a rough guide to a discussion, and as concrete information arises from the discussion, it can be entered onto the questionnaire. Alternatively, notes can be kept of interviews (whether person-to-person or group interviews) and pertinent information can be transferred to the questionnaire at a later stage. Or, and this is most usual, the questionnaire is used directly during a formal interview, and its structure strictly followed, point for point.

No matter which way a questionnaire is used, its design is of great importance to the success of information gathering, and a number of important principles apply:

- Content

This refers to the actual variables to be recorded. They will have been decided during the design stage of the information system, and must be kept to a minimum.

- *Time*

The length of the interview (which is directly determined by the number of variables to be recorded) must be short. 15 minutes is a practical guideline, shorter is better. When doing complex surveys (eg. Rapid Appraisals), interviews may become longer, but under those circumstances, anything longer than one hour is excessive.

- *User-friendly*

The questionnaire layout must be clear and logical so that the interviewer follows a logical sequence down the page from start to finish. Likewise, it must provide a logical sequence for the data entry clerk to follow when transferring data from the questionnaire to the database. It must also be clear and legible. Certain parts of the questionnaire may contain comments or information not intended for the database - these should be clearly marked.

- *Self-contained*

The form must be self-contained in that all necessary information is contained on it - district, date, details of interviewer, name of place, disease information etc.

- *Coding*

Where possible, information should be coded on the form to simplify and accelerate data input. If the code for a particular district is a set of letters, the field worker should enter his district's letters on the form - or they could be pre-entered before a field visit is undertaken. Species, such as "Bovine" could be ticked off in an appropriate "check box" on the form. Nonetheless, on-form coding should be approached with care. If check boxes for every conceivable alternative of every variable are provide on the form, it will become complex and possibly difficult to read and complete - perhaps leading to the wrong boxes being checked, or even omitted. Dealing with purely "veterinary" information means that it is often best given in narrative form and then encoded at input level - for example, issues such as clinical signs or post-mortem lesions. Giving a few alternative signs on a form will lead to all syndromes reported having very similar appearances. Such a form of information collection could also have the effect of being a set of leading questions, in which farmers are lead to describe a particular condition.

- Consider the possible effects of the following interview:

    "Did your animals show discharges and diarrhoea before death?"

- As opposed to:

    "Please describe all abnormal signs you noticed before your animals died."

The first question is clearly leading, and if animals did not show clinical signs within the narrow range given, confusion will result. Either the stock owner will assent to the few symptoms given, even if they were not seen (after all, his animals *did* die) or he may be reluctant to co-operate further. The interviewer will simply record what he is told, blissfully unaware of whether it is valid or not, and garbage will enter the system.

The second question allows a full description of what really happened, and the interviewer will get closer to the truth. Instead of being forced to fit all diseases seen into what will perforce be narrow sets of clinical signs, it will be possible to identify a wider range of diseases. It will thus be possible to get early warning of new - and hitherto unknown - diseases in the area.

Clinical signs and post-mortem lesions are best left as open as possible so that farmers have a free reign to describe exactly what they saw, and are not limited by a few choices on a questionnaire. In such cases, encoding can be done at the level of computerisation, where a full list of codes to cover every symptom and lesion can be kept, and used during input.

- Presentation

Issues such as paper size and quality, clarity of printing and size of spaces for recording answers deserve careful consideration. A smart, simple questionnaire will further ensure good quality information. Shoddy, overcrowded and complex forms will be completed in a shoddy manner.

Questionnaires should be so designed as to accommodate all diseases, not custom-made to suit just one. Expecting field workers to carry a variety of questionnaires, each for use with a different disease is wasteful of resources and will only cause confusion. (The same, incidentally, goes for the database - creating a separate information system for each disease is senseless. The entire system should be broad-based enough and robust enough to cope with any eventuality. Anything less than this reflects poor system design).

A few specimen questionnaires are given at the end of this manual as examples.

Start-up hints

Using questionnaires for the first time means a few things. First of all, an instruction manual should be prepared, explaining the questionnaire in greater detail. The aims of the questionnaire should be summarised. What is required under each data item (in logical order) should be explained.

Once this has been done, a number of the field workers who will be using the questionnaire should be trained in its use. A briefing on the contents of the questionnaire and how best to put the questions should be given first, and then the workers should use role-playing techniques to test their abilities among themselves. A field test is then carried out, with a senior staff member (preferably the questionnaire designer) accompanying each field worker for the first interview. Each worker is then allowed to do a few further interviews on his own.

After this exercise, the response of the field workers is evaluated, and the first data are examined in order to determine shortcomings with the questionnaire and modify it if necessary.

Databases

Databases, in their most general sense, are simply a means of storing data - whether it be on a computer or on a tabulation sheet, in a card index system or in a ledger. In recent times, however, the word "database" has almost become synonymous with "computer". Computers were, in fact originally conceived as high-speed data storage and retrieval mechanisms.

As computers are evolving at such a frightening speed, no attempt will be made to suggest specifications in this manual. Prospective users should consult with a number of vendors in order to gauge trends and make intelligent purchases.

Functions

Database software is generally able to store most types of data - whether as numeric or non-numeric variables, sort data, and retrieve specific items or subsets of data in response to user queries. Data files, or specific subsets, can also be exported into spreadsheet programmes for graphic analysis, and where data are georeferenced, can be introduced into GIS software to be visualised as maps.

As mentioned earlier, it is important to distinguish between data on questionnaires that are destined for computerisation and those that are not (eg. specific comments from field staff to their supervising veterinarian, or information cattle movements that needs to be followed up), and also to take note of the fact that certain information, while it must be computerised, will need action before it even reaches the computer (eg. a suspicion of a new disease outbreak).

Software

Various database programmes are currently available, and while these may change in the future, they can probably (at the time of writing) be divided into three broad categories:

- Software for small business (and therefore for relatively small datasets) -eg. Microsoft Access.

- "Middleweight" software for medium-sized databases of all types - eg. Microsoft Visual FoxPro, Borland Visual dBase and Borland Paradox.

- Software for large-scale databases (often used by banks, large companies, government ministries, international organisations) - Oracle, Sybase.

No blanket recommendation can be made here regarding the "best" software to use, and the above can be taken as examples only. Software requirements will vary from system to system, and obviously according to data volumes collected. What is important is ensure that the hardware (ie. the computer) has the capacity to run the chosen software, and the system overall can cope with the input volume and the outputs required.

What also needs mentioning is that there are some more or less custom-made software packages available for epidemiological data storage and analysis. Some of these packages are old and most have very limited capacities.

Database software is normally good for storage, quick sorting and retrieval of data, and small statistical manipulations (eg. range, mean, std deviation) are sometimes possible. In order to carry out advanced data analysis, spreadsheet packages (eg. MS Excel, Corel Quattro-Pro) and statistics packages are needed (eg. StatGraphics, Kwikstat, Epi-Info). For spatial analysis, one moves into the advanced world of Geographic Information Systems (eg. ArcView, MapInfo).

File structures

Information is stored on computer in entities known as "files". Naming of files, and what goes into them (ie. their structure) is the prerogative of the user.

Database files are structured, with each observation (in our case, the equivalent of a questionnaire) recorded in the file as a "record". The variables in each record (eg. locality name, animal species, number sick, etc) are known as "fields." A group of records with a homogenous structure, and stored together, is known as a table.

There are different types of variables, and the software will handle each type differently - for example, a place name would be stored as a "character" variable, and the programme would be able, for example, to sort them alphabetically. The number of animals reported dead in an outbreak would be stored as a "numeric" variable, and calculations could be performed upon it. Variables and their types must be defined during database design, and must exactly follow the structure of the questionnaire.

As this is not a manual on database software, there will be no further discussion of software at this stage. Enough information on databases is available elsewhere.

Coding

As part of database planning, it is essential to choose a set of codes for each variable before the database is launched. For example, one disease may have many names, such as blackleg, black quarter, or quarter evil. Which of these to use in the database? It would be preferable to type in a standard code for the disease, such as BQ (or some other suitable, but recognisable, code). The data entry clerk could be supplied with a "look-up table" (which may be programmemed into the computer, or kept in a separate manual), look up one of the synonyms, and enter the correct code. Likewise, when it comes to symptoms, "drooling" and "salivation" might be encoded as SALIV.

Encoding means that information can easily be retrieved. When one wants to enquire about black quarter, it would not be necessary to ask separately about each of the three synonyms in order to get a full picture of the disease - one query using the code "BQ" would immediately render all the information available to the enquirer.

Data input staff soon become very familiar with the most common codes and after initial "teething" periods, will be able to enter the correct codes for most variables - districts, species, diseases, clinical signs, etc, almost without thinking.

Ease of input

Making inputs into the database must be a simple operation. The "user interface" through which the input staff have to work needs to be simple and friendly. Typing into a template and having on-line assistance available is a great help, and the order of input of variables must follow the order of the questionnaire. Having an easy-to-read manual written to help data entry clerks is ideal, and of course, training is essential. Data entry staff must also be chosen for their speed and accuracy, and their ability to cope with monotonous, repetitive work.

Querying the database

Most queries will be fairly simple, and most modern software has "query builders" built in which the user can employ in analysing data. Queries usually take the form of something like "list all the foci of pasteurellosis in bovines in district x for the month of June" or "calculate the sum of all CBPP cases diagnosed during the year."

Exactly how to formulate queries will be described in the software manual, and on-line help and hints are usually available within programmes. It is important that epidemiologists perform a standard set of queries very regularly (say each month) for reporting purposes. Having a set of standard outputs and analyses keeps field staff up and management alike up to date with the disease situation in the country, and helps foster confidence in the system.

Data quality control

Although data control has been mentioned earlier, it deserves further treatment at this point as a separate entity.

Data quality control is an integral part of information management. As has been made clear elsewhere in this manual, it is a fatal mistake to assume that all data entering a system are good data.

Data move from the field to the district office to database input. The more checks are conducted before input, the better. If a problem is detected while a piece of information is still relatively near to its source, it can be followed up and corrected with relative ease, the further data move from their origin, the more difficult - and costly - corrections become.

Checking levels and what is checked are as follows:

In the field:

Careful questioning of the farmer to capture a true reflection of epidemiological information. Leading questions should be avoided. If information comes from farmer recall, it may be worthwhile to cross-check information with other family members or in-contact farmers.

At the district office:

Completed questionnaires are evaluated for legibility, correctness (eg. place names, code usage) accuracy and internal logic. What is written must, in other words be clear, neat and make sense. Where a query arises, the district supervisor (preferably a veterinarian) must first contact the interviewer concerned to clarify the issue with him. If necessary, and if possible, a return should be made to the original data source (the farmer) to follow up. Not only is it easier (nearer) to do this while still at field level; it is also possible to recapture information while it is still within reasonable recall and important details are not yet forgotten.

At the epidemiology unit

The data entry clerks will detect - and complain about - poor handwriting. The epidemiologist will further do spot checks on individual questionnaires before data entry, and also cross-check data entered onto the database with the questionnaires from which the data came on a random basis.

Data input staff will need good training and careful monitoring. It essential that data typists do not sit in front of computers for extended periods, as this leads to physical tiredness, eye and mental fatigue and a lack of concentration. Where possible, data entry should be interspersed with other tasks, such as the sorting and filing of questionnaires, doing data backups, sending enquiries to the field about data quality, etc.

A very important task of the epidemiologist, mentioned only in passing thus far, is the detection of fabricated data. It is a painful truth that some field workers will not always visit each place on their visiting programmes, but may simply sit at home and complete questionnaires in their easy chairs. Discovering such data is not easy, but a few pointers might help. It is helpful to carry a preliminary analysis of data and look for tendencies. First, simply view recently entered data in its "raw" form in the table, and then carry out a few simple statistical procedures, such as calculation of range, mean, standard deviation, construct histograms, view data spatially with a GIS. Look for the following:

- repetition of the same, or similar values (eg. herd sizes, or numbers of animals affected by a particular disease).

- variables having a small standard deviation, with many values clustered around the mean.

- a very homogenous disease/clinical signs pattern in a particular area.

- many values ending in zeros or fives.

- herd size distributions that are vastly different in adjacent and very similar areas.

- many observations of herd inspections with little or ancillary information given on the questionnaires (eg. questions on clinical signs or pasture conditions may be unanswered).

- details given for a visit to a particular place may be identical to another visit to the same place six months previously, ie. the previous visit's questionnaire was copied.

- a particular disease being widespread in one worker's area while being absent from an adjacent area where prevailing conditions are very similar.

All of the above are reasons to be suspicious about data. Where there is a pattern of repetition in a particular worker's information, then his data are suspect. Where there are vast disparities between data of two adjacent field workers' areas, it will be difficult to say exactly which of the two is at fault. In general, however, it may be necessary to send an independent team into the field to conduct random inspections in the areas from which devious data have come as a verification study. Results can be compared afterward. Where it is obvious that a field worker has fabricated data, severe disciplinary steps must be taken.

Needless to say, field management of veterinary staff remains an important aspect of basic management, not just data management. Staff must work according to fixed programmes, and spot checks must be made by supervisors from time to time to ensure that they are actually "on programme."

Errors need not only be the result of fabrication, though. Biases in data can arise for other reasons, and epidemiologists must be aware of these. Routine surveillance is very often not randomised, but pre-programmed, and anomalies may arise:

- field workers might use motor vehicles and not always reach more remote areas. This may confine field work to areas near main roads where richer farmers often live. Such farmers usually have larger herds and flocks, and use more medicines and vaccines - with a correspondingly lower disease incidence.

- field workers are usually male. For various reasons associated with personal prejudice or cultural taboos, they will not interview women, and so gain inaccurate data on animal species with which women usually work, eg. poultry and small ruminants.

Even where surveys are randomised, errors will creep in. If livestock numbers are incorrectly estimated, serum sampling tubes may be too few, resulting in unrealistically small sample sizes. Sampling animals of unknown vaccination history may result in the detection of vaccine titres during sero-surveillance. Farmers may lie about what diseases their animals have had.

Data input staff may quite literally have a bad day and miss the typing-in of a batch of data forms - or forms may get lost in the post, leaving a "hole" in the database.

Lists of what can go wrong are endless and very depressing, but can be minimised through:

- thorough staff training (at field and headquarters level)

- creating strong farmer awareness and gaining their co-operation

- good planning of data collection, routine surveillance and special surveys

- enforcing strong discipline amongst staff

- having a vigilant epidemiologist

Verification

Verification has been mentioned already, but it bears repeating.

Giving feedback to the field in the form of analysed data regular reports is a good way of seeing whether trends registered in the database are a good reflection of trends on the ground. Another tactic - and this can be expensive - is to send each field veterinarian a monthly printout of all data entered from his district during the preceding month for him to inspect, correct and return to the epidemiology unit. In this way, records that were incorrectly entered can be corrected, and should the veterinarian wish to update some information on particular incident, he has the opportunity to do so. If this is too expensive, sending each veterinarian a six-monthly summary of his district's data may be a more viable option.

Visits by epidemiology unit staff to the field are an indispensable means of maintaining contact, and an opportunity for on-the-spot validation studies.

Feedback

The importance of feedback has thus far been mentioned several times. It maintains the chain of communication and ensures interest on the part of field staff. The question is, how?

Regular reports giving summaries of the disease status in various parts of the country are probably ideal. Such reports must be clear and interesting, well illustrated with graphs, maps and tables. Veterinarians must be encouraged to comment on such reports, write "letters to the editor" and contribute short articles on interesting cases. A lively rapport between the epidemiology unit and the field is certain to keep the information system alive, while at the same time ensuring that all field staff are kept well informed. Part and parcel of this communication will be regular meetings between district vets and their field staff to discuss the contents of such regular reports. It is of the utmost importance that this feedback reach the people who collect the data on the ground. They must be made to feel part of a team.

It is a good idea, as mentioned in the previous section to send each district - or even, where practically possible, each staff member a short summary of their reporting every six months. A short table giving disease totals together with one or two illustrative graphs is sufficient for each person to know that his data area received and appreciated. It also gives each person a "snapshot" of the situation in his area.

The role of GIS

GIS stands for Geographic Information System. A GIS is an automated (ie. computerised) system for the input, storage, analysis and output (viewing) of spatial information. Various software packages have been developed for the visualisation of geographically referenced data, all them resource-hungry, all of them expensive, and, for the epidemiologist, usually indispensable. In fact, running a veterinary information system without some kind of a mapping system – even a manual one – would be akin to trying to run a motor car without a speedometer or a fuel gauge.

The main advantage of GIS software is not just that the user is enabled to see how a disease is distributed geographically, but also that an animal disease can be viewed against other information - for example, rainfall maps, vegetation maps, rivers, and so on. The disease presence can then be related to other factors and more easily appreciated visually.

Georeferencing data

Using disease data within a GIS means that every observation of disease recorded in the disease database must be georeferenced (in other words, must be accompanied by latitude and longitude values or some other grid reference recognised by the software).

There are two main ways of handling this, each of which has advantages and disadvantages. One is to add georeferences to each report (ie. each questionnaire must have a place where georeferences can be filled in). The other method is to have a "master file" built into the computer database where the computer (automatically) or the input clerk (manually) can "look up" the latitude/longitude values and add them to the records.

Georeferences on the questionnaire

This can be done in a number of ways. Each field worker can be given a standard list of all georeferences for the places in his area of work, and can add to the data forms as he goes along, or he could look them up on his return to his district base and add them there. Alternatively, someone else at the district office could fill them in once the forms have been handed in, which might be preferable, as many field workers (especially those with lower educational levels) might not understand the principles involved, or might make too many errors. The district veterinarian would have to check the co-ordinates before sending the forms away for computerisation, but obviously would not be able to check everything in detail.

Getting georeferences from a computer table

This would entail having a database table containing the names and geographic co-ordinates of every place in the country that could conceivably be visited by field staff. From that point, things could happen in one of two ways:

The data entry clerk would enter the details from the lookup table into the main database each time an observation is entered. This poses some problems. Should the place name perchance not be in the lookup table, there would be no easy way to quickly ascertain the co-ordinates. The same would apply if the place name were misspelled on the questionnaire (hopefully a thorough check at district level would have obviated that possibility), or if place names had changed (as they sometimes do in traditional parts of Africa, for example). To make matters worse, one sometimes finds places in the same country and even the same area with the same names, giving rise to the question of which one is referred to on the data form.

The other possibility is to have software which scans the data entries and the lookup table systematically, and then enters the georeferences automatically after cross-matching place names in the disease data table with place names in the lookup table or master file. The same problems noted above for manual georeference entry would apply for such automatic entry.

Both concepts of georeference entry into the database - either at field level or at the computer level, are fraught with problems, and there are no easy solutions. Each country and system designer would have to cope with the issue in the way best suited to their circumstances.

Using the GIS

Nothing much will be said about use of GIS software, and the reader is advised to consult relevant literature on the subject. The prospective user must consult thoroughly before purchasing such software, bearing in mind the following points:

- the software must be compatible with the computer system in use. GIS programmes are usually resource-hungry, requiring much disk space, operating memory and fast processors. It may be necessary to upgrade an older computer system in order to accommodate modern GIS programmes.

- the GIS software must be compatible with the database system in use. The GIS treats different kinds of data as "layers" and essentially, disease data would be imported into the mapping system as a layer. It must first be ascertained whether the database format in use in the epidemiology unit can be "read" by the GIS; the next is to ensure that the manner in which the georeferences are stored can be read by the GIS. It may be necessary, for example, to convert degrees, minutes and seconds into decimal degrees (where, for example, 30° 30' 30" would be read as 30.5 degrees) before importing the database file into the GIS, or the GIS may do it automatically.

- there must be ready maintenance for the GIS software within easy reach, and it should be easy to acquire important layers (roads, weather data, etc) locally. Usually, GIS programmes when purchased, come with a world map containing little more than country borders and the grid references for capital cities. More details have to be purchased, begged, borrowed or stolen elsewhere.

- training and other support should also be available. GIS software, while having many advantages, and being important in good epidemiological practice, is notoriously difficult to use. The importance of good training cannot be over-emphasised.

Motivating and training field staff

Field staff must be carefully chosen and well-trained. Farmers are usually willing to part with information when they feel that field staff are intelligent, trustworthy and can offer something in return. Field staff should be able to offer advice on matters related to animal health, and should also be able to carry out "first aid" treatments should they encounter sick animals during the course of their rounds. Treatments need not necessarily be for free, but the service should be available. They should also be well-trained in questionnaire usage.

The ability to handle animals well, take blood samples competently and to interact with people are also essential prerequisites.

The same principles apply when using "outsiders" to collect information. There is a strong tendency to make use of Community Animal Health Workers or "barefoot vets" from the private sector as gatherers of information in the field. They are interviewed periodically and all disease information is transferred to questionnaires for computerisation. It should not necessarily be assumed that such people have all the training that they need. They too will have to be trained in certain basics before being used as trusted sources of information.

Basic training for livestock inspectors or community animal health workers

The kind of subjects that might be covered in such training (which must have a strong practical component) would include:

- The very basic principles of anatomy and physiology of the domestic animals in the area.
- Principles of nutrition and pasture ecology.
- Animal diseases of local importance: clinical and post mortem signs, epidemiology, prevention, treatment.
- Applying first aid, the use of basic veterinary medicines (wound treatments, dips, anthelmintics, antibiotics, trypanocides, babesiacides, vaccines, care and storage of medicines and vaccines, use and care of syringes, etc).
- The basic principles of sero-surveillance campaigns - how to draw blood, store sera, etc.
- Questionnaire usage, information recording and interview technique as appropriate.
- All teaching should be illustrated with colour slides and/or posters, and adequate practical work under local conditions is all-important.

Training should not be conducted such that all subjects are dealt with in one course. The course should be divided into modules, between which the workers will return to the field and apply their knowledge in practice. The teaching should be re-inforced with frequent revisions. Evaluations should be practical rather than in the form of written examinations.

While the training above is aimed at lay persons, it should not be forgotten that veterinarians will also need training is questionnaire use.

Logistics

Backing up field staff with sufficient supplies is basic to their functioning. Field staff who are undersupplied with their necessities will become frustrated and discouraged and will not function. The following issues must be considered:

- regular pay and access to food and clothing supplies if the staff are on the official payroll.

- transport in the field. Vehicles and motorcycles will require fuel, regular servicing and a supply of spare parts.

- protective clothing. There should be a regular issue of overalls and appropriate footwear.

- camping equipment should be available, especially for the rainy season.

- a plentiful supply of questionnaires, carbon paper (to make duplicate copies), pens, pencils and clipboards is essential.

- basic medicine kits with a few essential stock remedies, needles and syringes.

- other supplies, such as serum collection tubes, labels, markers, ear-tags, vaccines, cold boxes, and so on, must be readily available at the appropriate times.

Awareness creation among decision makers

Many veterinarians in senior positions are currently not familiar with modern information systems development, and may have false expectations of information systems. They may even be suspicious of them, or simply discount them.

There are those who treat computers with contempt after having had one or two bad experiences with them, or who simply do not understand them. Others, on the other hand, may be over-enthusiastic, and expect too much. Some may think that installing a computer and some database software will create an information avalanche that will enable easy decision-making overnight. The latter group will suffer the most disillusionment when they discover that implementing an information system is a slow and painstaking process, and that the first information to come out of it is untrustworthy.

Having a computer system will not:

- Automatically improve information collection or quality. It may provide an impetus in this direction, but will not do so of itself.
- Provide instant disease status information within a few days of installation. Getting information into a system is a long process, and upgrading the quality of information

to make it reliable, is an even longer process. It will take one to two years or perhaps longer before outputs are intelligible and usable.
- Replace a good epidemiologist and common sense.

Having a computer system will:

- Take time to plan, install and implement.
- Have a lot of teething problems.
- Bring about cost savings in some areas. Blanket disease control campaigns are the norm in many countries. Having good disease data will show what diseases are present where, and what their incidence levels are. Control mechanisms will then be implemented more selectively and only in the areas where needed. It is a fact that, until recently, many African countries were still carrying out huge annual vaccination campaigns against rinderpest unnecessarily, simply because they had not quantified the threat and correctly identified the areas where it existed.
- Enable the monitoring of progress with disease control efforts, provided that consistent, accurate reliable data are being collected.
- Require a lot more headquarters-field liaison, and giving large quantities of feedback and encouragement.
- Cause management staff to appreciate field personnel a lot more and build valuable relationships and *esprit de corps*.
- Make decision making on disease management much easier - once the system is properly running.

Computer-analysed data form part of the information that goes into veterinary decision-making processes, but only a part. All planning must be done against a background of knowledge of staff capabilities, budgetary constraints, cultural values and traditions, and prevailing government policy. Decisions must be holistic and take all of reality into account, and not just the slice of it that comes from a computer.

Getting a system started

Leaving this section until this late in the manual has been deliberate. Having an overview of what a veterinary surveillance system will entail is essential before trying to design and implement one. Some ground has already been covered in previous pages, but some aspects still need discussion.

- Agreeing on the need for systematic data collection and analysis is an essential first step, that will require intense discussion between all stakeholders - management, the epidemiologist, field staff and laboratory staff.

- Designing the system, taking into account any system that already exists, is the next step. Crucial decisions must be made regarding data sources, inputs and outputs.

- Database design is the next step, together with software customisation and questionnaire design. Several questionnaires may need to be designed according to information sources-visual surveillance, abattoir surveillance, and so on.

- The next stage is field testing. It would be most practical to do a few pilot runs in two or three selected areas, completing questionnaires, following the information flow into the computer, and then doing some trial analyses. Shortcomings can be identified and corrected.

- Then all veterinarians will have to be informed and trained in implementing the system, and they in turn will need to train their field staff.

- The system is then implemented. Data flow and quality will have to be intensely and carefully monitored in order to make as many improvements as possible. It is important that both management and field staff be informed of what is happening every step of the way. If left in the dark, suspicions will develop, and enthusiasm and support will wane.

- All in all, it will take one to two years from conception to implementation. Allowing for some hiccups along the way, another year or two for the system to mature enough to produce "research quality" data.

- Bear in mind that no information system is ever static. It will continue to evolve and grow as needs change and users become more sophisticated.

Using surveillance data as a management tool

It is not the intention here to write a textbook on veterinary epidemiology, but rather to give few pointers. From the point of view of an epidemiologist, having a strong flow of "analysable" data can be very exciting. The trick is to make good use of it. First and foremost, it must be remembered that an information system is a management tool. Using information from a system for research and retrospective studies may be exciting, but day-to-day management is the aim.

Regular preparation of month-by-month incidence graphs of the main diseases can be very informative. Doing such work for one or two years may reveal important seasonal tendencies, particularly as far as vector-borne diseases are concerned, but possibly with others, as well. This may give good indicators as the planning of official strategic controls or regular reminders to farmers.

Longitudinal studies will also be of value in monitoring progress with eradication efforts, deciding when best to enter an OIE pathway, or to change from visual surveillance for a particular disease to sero-surveillance or abattoir surveillance.

Spatial analyses using a GIS are extremely useful for monitoring disease spread, and for noting the association a disease may have with weather conditions, ecological zones or geographic features such as rivers or roads. Areas under particular threat can be noticed early in the development of a disease, enabling the more rational deployment of resources. Planning for staff distribution, transport arrangements and vaccine purchases is facilitated.

Long-term studies of disease data will also reveal cyclical tendencies, association with long-term climate changes, and so on. It may even be possible to build reliable models of some diseases which enable predictions of spread to be made with greater accuracy.

An important fact about disease information systems is the ability to link them with economic data, and make inferences regarding economic impacts of diseases and the costs and benefits of control measures. Computer software can then be harnessed for building reliable "what-if?" scenarios and allowing an intelligent choice of various control options to be made.

FAO involvement in information and surveillance systems development for Transboundary Animal Diseases

The preparation of this manual is testimony of FAO's commitment to assist developing countries with development of their own early warning systems. Via the EMPRES programme, FAO is involved at national, regional and global level with the development of disease early warning systems. The ultimate vision is a global network, linking member countries in an information network that will enable rapid disease reporting, and quick dissemination of information.

This network will be a part of the Global Early Warning System (GEWS) being established by FAO to cover all possible pests, diseases and natural disasters.

EMPRES is currently involved in the development of a three-tiered information system which will gather, process and disseminate information. It is essentially a computerised system, to be known as the Transboundary Animal Disease Information system (TADInfo). This will consist of three different software modules: TADInfo National, TADInfo Regional and TADInfo Global.

For countries lacking properly developed epidemiological software, TADInfo National will be available free of charge. Through the well-established TCP system, FAO will be able to assist with information system development and software installation. TADInfo National is designed to feed information upwards to TADInfo Regional, which will be installed at the level of collaborating regional organisations or projects (such as PARC, SADC or PANAFTOSA) or at regional/subregional FAO offices. Where countries already use their own internally developed software, provision can be made for feeding-in of information from these systems.

Finally, the regional TADInfo modules will feed information to the global module, located in FAO headquarters.

Basically, the functions of the different modules will be:

- at national level: storage and analysis of disease information to facilitate local decision-making.

- at regional level: regional early warning, regional support and co-ordination.

- at global level: risk modelling, trend monitoring and global early warning.

FAO will also take the initiative of organising regional workshops for veterinary epidemiologists to share and disseminate information on disease surveillance.

At the Annual OIE General Session, held in Paris, France in May 1998, FAO was given the mandate, along with OIE and WHO, to build a global information system for disease early warning. This resolution (no. XIII of the 66th General Session) supports an earlier mandate from the 1996 World Food Summit.

The FAO is fully committed to this ideal, and will continue to work towards it via:

Software (TADInfo) development;
In-country support in the form of TCPs;
Regional workshops;
The EMPRES Livestock Website on the Internet;
and electronic mail discussion groups.

Interested CVOs and national epidemiologists should contact their nearest FAO office to enquire about the ways in which FAO can assist with the building of national and regional information systems.

Examples of questionnaires

Example of Report Form for use by Community Animal Workers/Animal Health Assistants

Name: .... **District:** .... **Year:** .... **Month:** ....

Village:		Disease	Species	# Cases	# Dead	Main sign
No. cattle						
No. sheep						
No. goats						
No. camels						
No. poultry						

Village:		Disease	Species	# Cases	# Dead	Main sign
No. cattle						
No. sheep						
No. goats						
No. camels						
No. poultry						

Village:		Disease	Species	# Cases	# Dead	Main sign
No. cattle						
No. sheep						
No. goats						
No. camels						
No. poultry						

Village:		Disease	Species	# Cases	# Dead	Main sign
No. cattle						
No. sheep						
No. goats						
No. camels						
No. poultry						

Village:		Disease	Species	# Cases	# Dead	Main sign
No. cattle						
No. sheep						
No. goats						
No. camels						
No. poultry						

Example of reporting form (passive surveillance) for use by veterinarians and technical-level field staff

Example Disease Report Form

Instructions:
One form is to be completed for each focus/incident of disease reported. The questionnaire is to be completed clearly and legibly, and the shaded areas **must** be filled in.

Province/Region (4-letter code)		District (6-letter code)	

Locality		Grid Reference	Lat		Long	

Date	Year		Month		Day		Farmer name	

Disease/Diagnosis		Differential Diagnosis	

Nature of Diagnosis	Suspected		Clinical		Smear		PM		Laboratory	

SPECIES: (Bov/Ov/Cap etc)		AFFECTED POPUL-ATION (mark the correct word)	SEX	AGE	SYSTEM	
			male	neonate	dairy	beef
NUMBER Cases (total affected)			female	juvenile	mixed	trad
			castrate	subadult	intensive	
NUMBER Dead			all	adult	extensive	
NUMBER At Risk			?	all	other	
			?	?		

MEASURES ADOPTED		MAIN CLIN. SIGNS	MAIN PM LESIONS	EPIDEMIOLOGY
Treatment				(source, rate of spread, vectors, reservoirs, sporadic, continuous etc)
Vaccination				
Dip				
Quarantine				
Other				
None				
?				

Details of reporting officer:

Surname, initials:		Position	VET	VET AUX/PARAVET	LAY

Alternative Specimen Report Form (passive surveillance)

Background information

Date		Farming system	
Reporting Officer		Comments and relevant background information	

Geographic information

Region		District		Locality	

Species affected

Species affected (check)	*Bovine*	*Ovine*	*Caprine*	*Porcine*	*Other (specify)*

Numbers involved

No. Cases		No. Deaths	
No. at Risk		No. Examined	

Categories most affected

Age category (check)	*neonate*	*juvenile*	*subadult*	*adult*	*all*		*unknown*
Sex category (check)	*male*	*female*	*neutered*	*both*	*unknown*		

Signs and lesions observed

Clinical signs	
Post-mortem lesions	

Actions implemented

Treatments (list)				
Other (check)	*Vaccination*	*Dip*	*Quarantine*	*Cordon*
Samples sent to (name lab)				
Date of submission		Type of sample/s		

Details of Diagnosis

Tentative Diagnosis		Differential Diagnosis	

Basis for diagnosis (check)	*Rumour*	*Clinical history*	*Clinical signs*	*Blood smear*	*Laboratory test*

Example of reporting form for use in sero-surveillance

SERO-SURVEILLANCE REPORT FORM

First part for use by field staff   Survey ID _____

Survey officer details

Category:	VET	AHI	Initials:		Date (dd/mm/yy):	

Farm / Locality Details

Province/ Region		District		Locality name	

Details and history of animals sampled

Species		Breed/Type		Sex category		M	F	Castr	A
Age category	Younger than wean		Older than wean		Adults		All		
Condition of animals	G	M	P	Condition of veld			G	M	P
Vaccinations past year				Diseases past year					
No. of serum samples taken									
Animals moved in from?				Animals moved to?					

Disease being surveyed _____

Second part for completion by laboratory staff

Lab. reference number:_____ Technician:_____ Veterinarian:_____

Disease:	
Test:	
No. negative:	
No. suspicious:	
No. positive:	
Remarks:	

Sensitivity: _____ Specificity: _____

Any comments to Epidemiology Unit:

Third part for completion by Epidemiology Unit staff

Date entered_____ Data entry clerk_____ Checked by_____

Name of database table_____ Date checked_____

Example of reporting form for use at abattoirs (laboratory results entered on the reverse of the form)

ABATTOIR /SLAUGHTER SLAB REPORT FORM

Instructions:

This form is completed when:
(1) Any transboundary/other notifiable disease is diagnosed (even if only one case)
(2) When a consignment has more than a 5-10% incidence of other diseases of importance as identified by the Department of Veterinary Services.
(3) Any sample is sent to the Laboratory for whatever reason.

Where two different conditions are diagnosed in the same consignment, two separate forms must be completed.

The reverse side of the form is to be filled in when a sample is submitted to a laboratory. the original must accompany the sample to the laboratory, and a duplicate must be sent to Head Office for computerisation.

The reference number refers to any numeric series of your own choice, eg. 002/1996. These numbers must follow one another successively on successive forms, and must not be abattoir consignment number, etc...

The shaded boxes *must* be filled in.

Date	Abattoir (abbreviation)	Officer initials (1st, 2nd & last)	Reference number	
Owner of Animals	Locality/Farm Name		Province/Region	District
Species	Condition suspected or diagnosed		Differential Diagnosis	
Indicate whether it was diagnosed:	Ante-Mortem		or	Post-Mortem
No. of animals in consignment:	No. affected		Age of affecteds (weeks, months, years, 2t, 3T, all ages)	
Sex of affected (M = male, F = female, B = both)		Other comments:		
If you conducted any tests, what were your findings:				
Please mark with an X if samples to lab:				

Reverse of abattoir and field disease report form:

DETAILS FOR SPECIMEN(S) – LABORATORY

Number & type of specimen(s):	Time collected (only for sensitive organisms):	In case of RABIES, was there any human contact: [Yes] [No] If Yes, how many people affected ....
	Examination(s) requested:	Owner's name on reverse of this form: Owner's address: Owner's tel. number:
	ID and reference number if from satellite laboratory:	If not official – does lab have permission to do extra test at owner's cost: [Yes] [No] Costing: [Official] [Post price list]

FOR LABORATORY USE ONLY						
Date samples received	Lab number	Number copies required			Distribution	
Sections	micro/path	path	chem tox	Referral centres (specify)	Add. examination decided upon	
	nutr	virol	serol			
Is this a follow-up report	Yes	No	Another report to follow		Yes	No

LAB RESULT (FREE FORMAT)

LABORATORY COMMENT TO FIELD VET:

PATHOLOGY

Blood smear:	Respiratory system:
Eggs per gram:	Central nervous system:
General:	Musculoskeletal system:
Body cavities:	Skin:
Gastrointestinal tract:	Other:
Liver:	Pathological diagnosis:
Urogenital system:	Aetiological diagnosis:
Circulatory system:	Differential diagnosis:
Lymphnodes:	

COMMENT/RECOMMENDATION:

Appendix I: Random sampling design

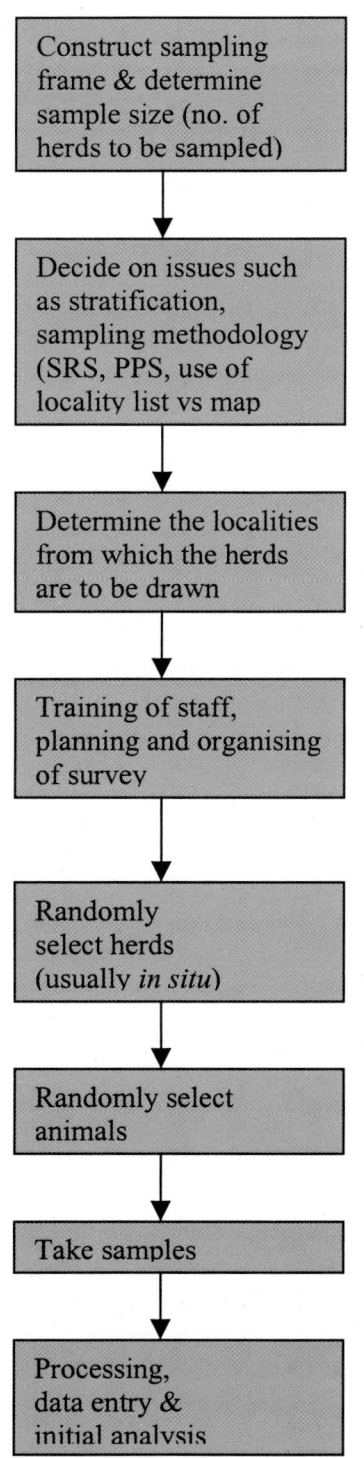

Construct sampling frame & determine sample size (no. of herds to be sampled)

Decide on issues such as stratification, sampling methodology (SRS, PPS, use of locality list vs map

Determine the localities from which the herds are to be drawn

Training of staff, planning and organising of survey

Randomly select herds (usually *in situ*)

Randomly select animals

Take samples

Processing, data entry & initial analysis

Sampling methods in randomised surveys

Conceptually, there are a number of steps involved in a disease survey. They are laid out below in a stepwise manner and will be explained in more detail later.

1. Sampling Frame

The construction of a sampling frame is the first step in the planning of a survey, and will be a reflection of "what question must this survey answer?" The sampling frame is a list of the "objects" in the sampling universe, giving the epidemiologist a catalogue or inventory from which to select the villages and herds which need to be sampled.

This is usually one of the most difficult and demanding parts of any survey exercise, as a surveillance effort will easily founder on a poorly designed sampling frame. If the sampling universe from which a sample is to be drawn is "all herds of cattle in district A", then it essential to have either a list of all the herds, or at least a list of all the places at which herds of cattle may be found. The completeness of the frame will obviously influence the representativeness of the sample.

Sampling frames can be drawn up from farmer address lists kept by extension officers, from population census records, maps of villages/cattle posts, or, in more sophisticated areas, telephone directories and post office address lists.

In areas where such information is unavailable, or which are inhabited by pastoral nomads, it is often only possible to make use of a large-scale map: the map is drawn into quadrants, each of which is assigned a number from 1 to *n*, and then quadrants are selected at random. These quadrants are then physically visited on the ground. This method is obviously far less secure than a proper sampling frame.

2. Sample size determination

Sample size depends on exactly what level of disease prevalence is to be detected, and at what level of confidence (in epidemiological work, a confidence level of 95% is the norm). The following formula may be used for populations > 1000:

$$n = \frac{(\log(1-\ ))}{[\log(1-\ d/N)]}$$

where n=sample size, =confidence level, d=estimated number of diseased, N=population size

As is now the case in most statistical tasks, the memorisation and manual usage of complex mathematical formulae is becoming virtually redundant, and there are many simple computer software packages available (some of them free of charge) which will perform these calculations with ease.

3. Stratification

Where a population of animals or livestock owners is extremely large, or spread over a number of different farming systems or distinct ecozones, it would be advisable to break the population into a series of smaller segments for the purpose of sampling. This process is known as stratification, and each new segment is known as a stratum. It is essential that the population within each stratum is as uniform as possible, thus ensuring more representative sampling. The various strata are treated as individual sampling universes wth their own sampling frames. While stratification effectively increases the overall number of samples taken, it also improves the overall quality of the sampling exercise. However, in order to keep costs to a minumum, it is advisable also to keep the number of strata in a single sampling exercise to a minimum – the criteria used for stratification should be such that no more than three strata are demarcated.

4. Methodology

The magnitude of most sampling exercises is usually such that a multistage sampling strategy is adopted. It is usually impossible to create, from the very first, a complete list of all cattle herds in a region and then choose them randomly. To compile a sampling frame of this size is usually too resource-intensive.

Sampling is then undertaken in two or more stages, for example:

(1) Draw up a list of places where herds are known to be kept (a primary sampling frame). Then choose the places to be sampled at random.

(2) Draw up a list of herds kept only at each chosen locality (secondary sampling frame). Then choose the herds at random.

Localities can be chosen (depending on the quality of the primary sampling frame) by one of three methods: Probabilities Proportional to Size (PPS); Constant Sampling Fraction (CSF) or from a map (by grid). These methods will be dealt with in turn below.

PPS method

Let us take an example where it is decided to sample a total of 15 herds. The designers determine that a minimum of 5 herds should be sampled in each locality. The sampling frame is of a high quality; ie. all the villages in the area are known, and the number of herds at each village is also known. The numbers of herds together with their villages are tabulated and cumulative totals worked out as shown below.

Village	No. herds	Cumulative	Random #
A	7	7	
B	8	15	13
C	10	25	
D	9	34	
E	15	49	49
F	7	56	51

Three random numbers are chosen, and the villages within which random numbers fall are the ones where the sampling exercise is carried out. A detailed sampling frame is then drawn up for each of the villages, and the primary sampling units (herds) chosen by simple random sampling.

CSF method

In the first stage, a number of posts would be chosen randomly, and for the second stage, a predetermined percentage of households at the selected posts would be chosen at random - eg. 20% of all households at the settlement. This method is ideal for transhumant peoples, where one cannot say with certainty beforehand how many people will be at each post. Upon arrival at a settlement, the enumerator will allocate each household a number and draw a number of them (equal to 20%) from a hat.

It is assumed that the (a) the total number of animals in the area is known and that (b) at least the various posts/settlements are known. In other words, a rudimentary sampling frame containing all known inhabited settlements has been drawn up. If prior calculation shows that the total number of animals to be sampled is roughly equal to, eg. 20% of the animals in the population, then 20% of each randomly sampled herd is bled. This method is not ideal, and is normally used only when there is uncertainty as to distribution of herds (eg. in situations of transhumance).

Random Geographic Co-ordinates

This method is used in areas populated by nomads, or where no sampling frame is available at all. It is the least reliable of the three methods described here. A map of the area to be surveyed is divided into squares of suitable size (5-10km blocks in real terms) and each square is allocated a number. The requisite number of squares (equivalent to the number of villages in the examples given above) are chosen using a random number table/random number generator. It is assumed that the number of herds to sampled at each point has already been decided; on the ground, this number of herds will be sampled within 5km radius of the physical centre of the square. An obvious disadvantage of this method is that travel might be undertaken to a chosen locality only to find the area uninhabited; in this case, a replacement locality is chosen at random as described above.

5. Choosing herds/animals once "on the ground"

The localities to be sampled are chosen by one of the methods described above. Actually choosing which herds will provide the candidate animals is a matter of cataloguing the herds at the sampling point and assigning each herd a number. Herds are then chosen using random numbers or literally drawing their assigned numbers from a hat.

Choosing animals to bleed is also not a major issue. It may be that the sampling frame calls for all animals in a particular age category; in which case no choice is involved. Where animals need to be chosen, those eligible for sampling can be assigned numbers and chosen randomly, or Linear Systematic sampling (LSS) can be used. With LSS, it is not necessary to number each individual animal, but the total must be known. The "sampling interval" (k) is calculated using the formula :

$k = N/n$ where N = the total number of animals available and n = the number required in the sample.

A random number (r) falling between one and k is then chosen. The sample then consists of every k^{th} animal. The animals are driven into a crush, and the first one sampled is r, then $r+k$, $r+2k$ etc.

Appendix II: A model framework for strengthening national and regional capabilities in disease surveillance (from the text adopted by EMPRES Expert Consultation 1999)

Introduction

Control and eradication of major epidemic diseases of livestock in any area of the world requires a coordinated regional approach. Countries in a region which have lower socio-economic standards are liable to fall behind their more developed neighbours in the area of animal disease control.

The majority of the population in most developing countries are involved in smallholder agriculture. This group also represents one of the poorest sectors of society. In addition to food and draft power, livestock represent an important savings system within the village economy. Livestock diseases cause enormous losses through death and decreased production. Strengthening the veterinary services of countries is an efficient, well targeted approach to improving the livelihood of the rural poor on a national, regional and global basis.

The key to a coordinated regional disease control program is the free exchange of reliable, compatible disease information between countries, and the harmonisation of reporting and disease control procedures. Encouraging a uniform approach to disease reporting and control programs throughout a region will help in control and eradication of diseases.

The objective of integrated control is to use a vertically integrated approach to improving the collection, management and use of animal health information for disease control. It achieves this by addressing weaknesses at every level of the information chain – from livestock owners to regional organisations. The long term aim is to support the development of veterinary services to enable them to successfully and sustainably control and eradicate major diseases of livestock. Examples of this are rinderpest in Africa and FMD in South America and South East Asia.

The rationale behind this approach is based on the current difficulty experienced by poorer countries in controlling emergency animal diseases and the presence of other possibly higher priority issues for government. Priority should be given to the establishment of successful, internally funded sustainable disease control programs within each country of a region. Such programs will produce significant benefits, not only through the control of the target disease, but also through establishing the infrastructure and skill-base amongst relevant staff. These skills can then be used to tackle other diseases of importance to the international community, which may be difficult and expensive to control. Commencing a disease eradication project without providing prior experience in the successful control of livestock diseases is likely to result in an expensive failure.

Objectives directed at ensuring an emergency response capability

The following are reasonably generic objectives which need to be met if a country is to have the capability to successfully deal with emergency animal diseases. By clearly defining objectives, the necessary outputs activities required to ensure an emergency response capability can be more effectively identified.

Objective 1:   *Improve the collection of animal health information*
Objective 2:   *Ensure Sustainable Laboratory Support*
Objective 3:   *Implement Information Management System*
Objective 4:   *Establish National and Regional Analysis and Reporting Systems*
Objective 5:   *Control Program Formulation, Implementation and Monitoring*

Outputs and Activities

In this section, the required outputs and activities are briefly summarised for each objective.

Objective 1:   Improve the collection of animal health information

Passive Surveillance

Improved disease reporting and specimen submission by livestock owners, village veterinary staff, district and provincial veterinary officers.

Passive surveillance gathers information through disease outbreak reporting and the submission of diagnostic specimens to veterinary laboratories. The level of under-reporting in passive surveillance systems means that the data collected is unrepresentative and unable to be used for developing control strategies, or addressing disease outbreaks. In countries where laboratory facilities are limited, the key personnel in the chain of reporting are the district officers who are responsible for submitting primary disease reports.

Training of provincial and district veterinary staff
Highly targeted training to district staff should be provided to equip them with the skills to carry out a disease outbreak investigation, recognise key transboundary diseases, restrain animals, collect specimens, collect disease history information and submit specimens to the laboratory. Training should be provided in a two-stage process, initially involving provincial staff. They should receive detailed training to develop the necessary technical skills as well as appropriate methods to pass on those skills to district staff (the "train the trainer" concept). The provincial staff can then be responsible for training district staff according to a plan which can be audited to ensure objectives are met. It is very important to provide basic training for para-veterinary staff, as they are often the only ones to have regular contact with farmers.

Provision of specimen collection kits
District staff need to be issued with basic sample collection kits (including restraint equipment, specimen collection equipment, transport containers and media, disinfectant etc), and pads of recording and laboratory submission forms.

Provision of ongoing support for district staff
After being trained, district staff need to be supported by provincial staff in carrying out field disease outbreak investigations, as they arise.

Monitoring staff activity
The activity of provincial and district staff in disease outbreak investigations, disease reporting and submission of specimens should be monitored with the assistance of an

information management system of some type, preferably computerised. Provinces and districts that appear to be failing to report disease and submit specimens can then be identified, problems and constraints investigated, and any necessary further training and support provided. Information management systems need to reflect both the business of the animal health authorities and existing information flows. Examples are the systems in place in Namibia, Laos and the Philippines (for FMD only).

Establishment of specimen transport and feedback systems
Systems for the effective transport of specimens to the laboratory, feedback to province, district and villages, and the sustainable maintenance of restraint equipment and submission materials should be in place and strengthened where required. To assist laboratories with feedback to the districts and villages, simple information sheets on disease control and prevention are needed for specific common diseases.

Continuing veterinary education for provincial and district staff
Provincial staff should be invited to attend periodic 'refresher courses' on commonly encountered diseases or issues, run by national counterparts, to strengthen field diagnostic skills and update knowledge on locally appropriate control or prevention options. They should be provided with training materials and required to present the same information to district staff at regular provincial meetings.

Public awareness campaigns for livestock owners and traders
As these persons are the first link in early warning of TADs, it is very important to devote considerable resources to public education and awareness. Encouraging the support of livestock owners in disease reporting can be achieved through the development of appropriate public awareness and education materials in the local language and at a level consistent with local education levels.

Establish links with village-level agricultural projects
Links should be established with agricultural development projects working at the village level (e.g. NGOs) to include this message in their work and distribute educational material.

Active Surveillance

Active surveillance to collect reliable, population-based information on key diseases, and to monitor the progress of disease control/eradication campaigns is an extremely useful activity to complement passive surveillance.

Comprehensive survey techniques have been developed by various international aid projects and a variety of survey manuals, software, and training course syllabi are available. These materials should be used as a basis to implement institutionalised, sustainable surveillance systems tailored to the needs of specific countries and the disease problems they are likely to encounter.

Training of provincial and district staff in survey techniques
Existing materials and techniques can be used to provide training to provincial and district staff in basic epidemiology, survey and random selection techniques.

Implementing field disease surveillance
Training should be centred around actual field surveillance exercises to give all staff an opportunity to practice and perfect their skills.

Development of a coordinated active surveillance program
In collaboration with national staff, a coordinated program of active surveillance should be established, targeting priority diseases. This would initially aim to provide baseline measures of disease incidence and antibody prevalence with a national coverage. To ensure the sustainability of the techniques, previously trained staff should be called upon to conduct regular surveys on priority issues as part of their normal responsibilities.

Use active surveillance to support disease control programs
Surveillance activities should be heavily emphasised in priority areas to support newly established or modified disease control programs.

Ancillary Data

Training a range of personnel in reporting and data collection techniques relevant to their responsibilities is vital to ensuring that ancillary data which supports disease control is properly recorded, analysed and reported.

Train personnel in the collection of ancillary data
A range of staff should receive basic training in the use of reporting forms for the collection of information of a variety of types. These include:

- Livestock movement checkpoint staff recording livestock movement data, and disease surveillance data;
- Vaccine production and distribution staff recording production and administration data,
- Vaccine teams recording vaccine administration data,
- Meat inspectors recording findings and producing reliable reports,
- District staff collecting village livestock population data.

Socio-economic Data

Train national-level staff in the collection of socio-economic data
National-level staff should receive training in the conduct of surveys to collect socio-economic data. This should be combined with active surveillance activities, and be aimed to support priority setting and control program formulation activities.

Objective 2:   Ensure sustainable laboratory support

A vital component of having the capability to manage emergency diseases is to have competent laboratory support. However, having a laboratory capability will only be fully effective where laboratory services are fully integrated into the overall surveillance and disease control programs. Where possible, training and program planning should include both field and laboratory personnel. This has been the approach in the Philippines in the FMD eradication program and has led to a greater understanding of mutual problems and more effective use of laboratory resources.

Effective laboratory support for field activities

Provision of specimens to national laboratories and international reference laboratories
Without a regular flow of specimens to these laboratories from the field, staff will not have an opportunity to perfect their skills, and little used tests may become unreliable. All field surveillance activities should feed specimens into national laboratories in a planned way which accounts for the capacity of the laboratories. Thus, the field surveillance effort must be designed so that it is fully integrated with laboratory capacity. National laboratories should also be made aware of the need to regularly send field isolates to reference laboratories for characterisation and serotyping.

Provision of diagnostic reagents to laboratories
In addition to maintaining staff skills, the sustainability of the diagnostic laboratories depends on a reliable supply of diagnostic reagents. A guaranteed supply of essential reagents and laboratory disposables must be available to support surveillance activities.

Development of systems for the sustainable local production of key diagnostic reagents
In some instances, it may be possible to produce some reagents locally within the laboratory. Others may have to be bought or imported. Reagents suitable for local production should be identified, and staff trained and systems set up for their sustainable production. The importance of standardising reagents and tests to international norms should be recognised.

Train laboratory staff in new diagnostic techniques as appropriate
Serological techniques such as ELISA have been developed to assist the diagnosis of many priority diseases. These require the provision of appropriate reagents and materials, and an ongoing access to training. For some priority diseases, additional simple and rapid tests exist. Staff should be trained in these techniques to broaden the range of diseases that can be handled at laboratories.

Objective 3:   Implement information management system

The main features of a useful information management system are that it is simple to use; inexpensive and quick to develop; able to handle a wide range of information related to animal health; can be modified locally to meet changing needs; and provides specialised epidemiological analytical procedures. With modern technology and a systematic approach to the analysis of business needs, systems can be quickly developed and implemented which meet the needs of all levels of animal health personnel and which are tailored to operate within the organisational structure of the country in question. A wide range of report formats can be incorporated including automated disease mapping where base maps are available.

Efficient management of animal health information

User needs analysis and database designs
Experience suggests that databases need to be specifically designed to work within the administrative and organisational structure of a particular country. However, if a modularised system can be developed, tailoring the system to meet the needs of specific countries is made much easier. Core modules are likely to require minor modification for use in different

countries, but there are likely to be country-specific needs which will require greater effort to develop.

Development and translation of users' manuals

Comprehensive users manuals should be developed and translated for each system. A core manual prepared in English could provide the basis for all manuals. This could be modified to take into account country differences, and then translated. Bilingual versions should be available in each country.

Training of staff in the use of systems

Inputs into information systems come from many different areas within the veterinary services of a country. Staff involved should all be trained in their roles and contributions to the system. A small team of national staff should be trained in the detailed operation of the system, including data entry staff, as well as national epidemiology staff involved in data analysis and reporting.

Phased implementation

Where required, systems should be implemented in a phased fashion, running in parallel with existing systems for some time, and gradually introducing more of the modules until the whole system is up and running. Where possible, implementation should be at least at provincial and national level.

Objective 4:   Establish National and Regional Analysis and Reporting Systems

Because of the ease of movement of livestock and diseases from one country to another, disease control requires a regional approach. National staff need to develop the skills to analyse data, and then be able to use the results to establish cooperative regional approaches to disease control.

Improved ability of national staff to analyse and interpret animal health information

Training of national staff in data analysis

National epidemiologists need to work alongside experienced personnel in the analysis of national disease information. On-the-job training should be provided through participating in the work. Sub-regional workshops for national staff of identified core countries should be conducted to provide more structured training in epidemiological data analysis and disease control program formulation.

Language training

English, French, and Spanish are the most common languages for animal health information systems. It is important that staff be competent in the language relevant for the region. If necessary, specific language training should be provided for staff. This will increase their ability to participate fully in regional meetings, prepare publications and reports, access the international literature and use many software programs.

Improved regional communication and coordination of disease control activities

Regional activities should be conducted in close collaboration with an international facilitator.

Establishment of regional disease outbreak database
A regional geo-referenced database should be established to facilitate collation and analysis of animal health information. Each contributing country would then have access to up-to-date information about the disease situation of their neighbours, to help prevent the cross-border spread of diseases.

Regional data analysis
Regional coordinators will be required to cooperate with national staff and regional organisations to carry out regional analysis of data, and establish an effective regional disease reporting system. Data collected through passive surveillance, active surveillance, socio-economic studies, and livestock movement records should be analysed and reported.

Country coordinators' meetings
Where regional programs are instituted, country coordinators and any counterparts need to remain in close consultation. In addition to correspondence, there should also be regular meetings, say every six months, rotating through each of the regional countries. These meetings will serve to share the experience in different countries, allow a better sharing of resources, and ensure continuing compatibility between systems.

Economic group member coordination meetings
Links should be established with formal trading group committees to institutionalise regional information sharing and disease control activities. In addition to working with formal committees, a series of technical meetings could be called to:
- develop a technically sound, comprehensive manual of standard definitions and rules for disease reporting and disease control for priority diseases in the region. These standards should be based closely on the OIE International Animal Health Code, and conform to the requirements of this code.
- develop standards for information exchange and reporting between countries in the region, including minimum datasets, exchange formats, geo-referencing systems etc.

Short-term attachments
Staff from regional participating countries could be involved in short-term attachments or exchanges to the veterinary services in different countries in the region. Epidemiologists from the more developed countries would have an opportunity to learn of the difficulties facing their less developed neighbours and have a chance to share their expertise. Less developed country staff would have a chance to examine the operation of information systems and disease control activities in the more developed countries.

Newsletter
If formulated as a series of regional projects, a newsletter may be useful to be distributed to all countries in the region, focusing on practical and technical aspects of disease control, and providing an informal channel of communication. The newsletter should also be a vehicle for exchange of information on disease investigations.

Objective 5:   Control Program Formulation, Implementation and Monitoring

In collaboration with expert consultants where required, national staff would use the data collected during field activities as the basis for the formulation and analysis of disease control options, and identification of preferred programs.

National disease control strategies

Training
Subregional technical training of national epidemiologists from participating countries would include both analysis of epidemiological data and use of the results for the formulation of disease control strategies.

Formulate disease control options
In collaboration with expert consultants, national staff would formulate a range of disease control options, identifying priority diseases, and possible appropriate control measures.

Evaluate options to identify optimal strategies
Supported by disease surveillance and socio-economic data, the control options should be evaluated and optimal strategies determined.

Effective disease control activities

Support the implementation of identified priority disease control activities
Within the structure of the national veterinary services, existing control activities may be modified, or new activities implemented, and provincial and district staff would use active surveillance techniques to monitor the effectiveness of these programs.

Personnel

The implementation of a program such as that described in Section 3 above would require development of a series regional of business plans and involve a reasonable number of personnel. In addition to an overall program manager, regional coordinators would be required as well as full-time in-country advisers. Regional coordinators should be veterinarians with experience in disease control in the specific region as well as project management experience. Each regional coordinator would be based in a convenient capital city within the region and would be responsible for overall project management, country coordinator support, and regional activities.

One country coordinator should be placed in each of the participating countries within a region, and be responsible for day to day running of project activities. The country coordinators should be veterinarians with an interest in epidemiology, good interpersonal and management skills, and cultural sensitivity. In particular they should have well developed training skills.

One key staff member should be identified within each participating country in a region to work as a counterpart to the country coordinator. The country coordinators' positions could be phased out after the first two years, with counterparts taking over full responsibilities.

Short term expert consultants may be required for a variety of tasks, including computer programming, development of publicity materials, economics, laboratory diagnostic techniques etc.

Potential Collaboration

Implementation of a program such as that described in would require the cooperation of a number of agencies. Potential donor agencies would need to be identified during the planning phase and the program developed with their collaboration

Main Budget Items

The main items which may need to be budgeted for include:

- Core project personnel
- Ongoing technical support to national veterinary services
- Training of provincial and district staff
- Support of field surveillance activities, and
- Supporting regional cooperation.

Training and personnel costs are therefore likely to make up a significant part of the budget.

Some specific items which will need to be considered in developing budgets include:

- Provincial staff training courses
- District staff training courses
- Ancillary staff training courses
- Active surveillance field activities
- Passive surveillance restraint and specimen collection equipment
- Vehicles
- Project personnel
- Office and Computer equipment
- Laboratory staff training and reagent support
- Regional exchanges and short-term attachments
- Regional meetings
- Travel
- Project management costs
- Administrative support costs

Activities and Outputs by Administrative Level

Regional	Participation in regional meetings Establishment of Standard Rules and Definitions for disease reporting and control Forging links with appropriate regional bodies and committees Institutionalising regional cooperation Regional analysis of disease, and livestock movement patterns Establishment of regional disease outbreak databases
Subregional	Harmonised disease surveillance and reporting systems Sharing of disease information for improved ability to prevent cross-border movement of animals
National	Improved passive surveillance systems Establishment of effective active surveillance systems Improved understanding of priority diseases Short-term attachments and exchanges between countries Development of structured disease control programs for priority diseases Support and development of laboratory capabilities
Provincial	Training in active and passive surveillance Improved skills in disease outbreak investigation and response
District	Training in active and passive surveillance Improved reporting of livestock demographics Improved reporting of livestock movement
Village	Increased awareness of the need to report and control diseases

Project Activity Schedule

The GANNT chart below outlines how a project to deliver the required outputs might be delivered.

Year	Year 1				Year 2				Year 3			
Quarter	1	2	3	4	1	2	3	4	1	2	3	4
Objective 1: Improve the collection of animal health information												
Output 1.1: Passive Surveillance												
Activity 1.1.1: Training of Provincial and district Veterinary staff		■	■	■	■	■	■					
Activity 1.1.2: Provision of specimen Collection Kits		■	■									
Activity 1.1.3: Provision of ongoing support for district staff					■	■	■	■	■	■	■	
Activity 1.1.4: Monitoring staff activity					■	■	■	■	■	■	■	■
Activity 1.1.5: Establishment of specimen transport and feedback systems	■											
Activity 1.1.6: Continuing veterinary education for provincial and district staff		■			■	■			■			
Activity 1.1.7: Public awareness campaigns for livestock owners		■	■									
Activity 1.1.8: Establish links with village level agricultural projects	■											
Output 1.2: Active Surveillance												
Activity 1.2.1: Training of provincial and district staff in survey techniques		■	■	■	■	■						
Activity 1.2.2: Implementing field disease surveillance		■	■	■	■	■	■		■	■	■	■
Activity 1.2.3: Development of a coordinated active surveillance programs			■									
Activity 1.2.4: Use active surveillance to support disease control programs									■	■	■	
Output 1.3: Ancillary Data												
Activity 1.3.1: Train veterinary staff in the collection of ancillary data	■	■	■									
Output 1.4: Socio-economic Data												
Activity 1.4.1: Train national staff in the collection of socio economic data		■	■	■	■							
Objective 2: Ensure Sustainable Laboratory Support												
Output 2.1: Effective Laboratory support for field activities												
Activity 2.1.1: Provision of specimens to national laboratories	■	■	■	■	■	■	■	■	■	■	■	■
Activity 2.1.2: Provision of diagnostic reagents		■	■	■	■	■	■	■	■	■	■	■

Activity	1	2	3	4	5	6	7	8	9	10	11	12	13	14
to laboratories		█	█	█	█	█	█	█	█	█	█	█		
Activity 2.1.3: Development of systems for the sustainable local production of key diagnostic reagents					█	█	█	█						
Activity 2.1.4: Train laboratory staff in new diagnostic techniques as appropriate					█	█	█							
Objective 3: Implement Information Management System														
Output 3.1: Efficient management of animal health information														
Activity 3.1.1: User needs analysis and database design	█													
Activity 3.1.2: Development and translation of users' manuals			█	█										
Activity 3.1.3: Training of staff in the use of the system				█	█	█								
Activity 3.1.4: Phased implementation					█	█	█	█	█	█	█	█	█	█
Objective 4: Establish National and Regional Analysis and Reporting System														
Output 4.1: Improved ability of national staff to analyse and interpret animal health information														
Activity 4.1.1: Training of national staff and data analysis		█	█	█	█	█	█	█	█	█	█	█	█	█
Activity 4.1.2: English language training	█	█	█	█	█	█	█	█	█	█	█	█	█	█
Output 4.2: Improved regional communication and coordination of disease control activities														
Activity 4.2.1: Establishment of regional disease outbreak database	█	█												
Activity 4.2.2: regional data analysis			█	█	█	█	█	█	█	█				
Activity 4.2.3: Country managers meetings		█			█			█		█		█		
Activity 4.2.4: Regional member coordination meetings				█			█			█		█		
Activity 4.2.5: Short term attachments			█	█	█	█	█	█	█	█	█	█		
Activity 4.2.6: News letter			█	█	█	█	█	█	█	█	█	█		
Objective 5: Control Program Formulation, Implementation and Monitoring														
Output 5.1: National disease control strategies														
Activity 5.1.1: Training			█	█	█	█	█	█	█	█	█	█		
Activity 5.1.2: Formulate disease control options					█	█	█							
Activity 5.1.3: Evaluate options to identify optimal strategies						█	█							
Output 5.2: Effective disease control activities														
Activity 5.2.1: Support the implementation of identified priority disease control activities							█	█	█	█	█	█		

For Further Reading

Anon *Using dBase IV* Borland, 1993

Casley, D & Lury, D *Data Collection in Developing Countries* ELBS (1987)

IAEA/FAO *Recommended procedures for disease and serological surveillance as part of the Global Rinderpest Eradication Programme (GREP)* IAEA (1994)

Last, J (Ed) *A Dictionary of Epidemiology* Oxford University Press (1995)

OIE *Epidemiological Information Systems* OIE Revue Sci et Tech March 1991

Pfeiffer, D *Veterinary Epidemiology – An Introduction* Massey University lecture notes (1998)

Poate, C.D. & Daplyn, P.F. *Data for Agrarian Development* Cambridge University Press (1993)

Schwabe, C et al *Epidemiology in Veterinary Practice* Lea and Febiger (1977)

Thrusfield, M *Veterinary Epidemiology (2nd Ed)* Blackwell Science (1995)

Wonnacott R, & Wonnacott, T *Statistics – discovering its power* John Wiley & Sons (1982)

FAO ANIMAL HEALTH MANUALS

1   Manual on the diagnosis of rinderpest, 1996
2   Manual on bovine spongiform encephalopathy, 1998
3   Epidemiology, diagnosis and control of helminth parasites of swine, 1998
4   Epidemiology, diagnosis and control of poultry parasites, 1998
5   Recognizing peste des petits ruminants – A field manual, 1999
6   Manual on the preparation of national animal disease emergency preparedness plans, 1999
7   Manual on the preparation of national rinderpest contingency plans, 1999

Availability: October 1999

The FAO Animal Health Manuals are available through FAO Sales Agents or directly from the Sales and Marketing Group, FAO, Viale delle Terme di Caracalla, 00100 Rome, Italy; fax (+39) 06 5705 3360; e-mail: publications-sales@fao.org

Sales and Marketing Group Information Division, FAO
Viale delle Terme di Caracalla, 00100 Rome, Italy
Tel.: +39 06 57051 – Fax: +39 06 5705 3360
E-mail: publications-sales@fao.org

WHERE TO PURCHASE FAO PUBLICATIONS LOCALLY
POINTS DE VENTE DES PUBLICATIONS DE LA FAO
PUNTOS DE VENTA DE PUBLICACIONES DE LA FAO

• ANGOLA
Empresa Nacional do Disco e de
Publicações, ENDIPU-U.E.E.
Rua Cirilo da Conceição Silva, Nº 7
C.P. Nº 1314-C, Luanda

• ARGENTINA
Librería Agropecuaria
Pasteur 743, 1028 Buenos Aires
World Publications S.A.
Av. Córdoba 1877, 1120 Buenos Aires
Tel./Fax: +5411 48158156
Correo eléctronico:
wpbooks@infovia.com.ar

• AUSTRALIA
Hunter Publications
PO Box 404, Abbotsford, Vic. 3067
Tel.: 61 3 9417 5361
Fax: 61 3 9419 7154
E-mail: jpdavies@ozemail.com.au

• AUSTRIA
Gerold Buch & Co.
Weihburggasse 26, 1010 Vienna

• BANGLADESH
Association of Development
Agencies in Bangladesh
House No. 1/3, Block F
Lalmatia, Dhaka 1207

• BELGIQUE
M.J. De Lannoy
202, avenue du Roi, B-1060 Bruxelles
CCP: 000-0808993-13
Mél.: jean.de.lannoy@infoboard.be

• BOLIVIA
Los Amigos del Libro
Av. Heroínas 311, Casilla 450
Cochabamba;
Mercado 1315, La Paz

• BOTSWANA
Botsalo Books (Pty) Ltd
PO Box 1532, Gaborone

• BRAZIL
Fundação Getúlio Vargas
Praia do Botafogo 190, C.P. 9052
Rio de Janeiro
Núcleo Editora da Universidade
Federal Fluminense
Rua Miguel de Frias 9
Icaraí-Niterói 24
220-000 Rio de Janeiro
Fundação da Universidade
Federal do Paraná - FUNPAR
Rua Alfredo Bufrem 140, 30º andar
80020-240 Curitiba

• CAMEROUN
CADDES
Centre Africain de Diffusion et
Développement Social
B.P. 7317, Douala Bassa
Tél.: + 237 43 37 83
Télécopie: +237 42 77 03

• CANADA
Renouf Publishing
1369 chemin Canotek Road, Unit 1
Ottawa, Ontario K1J 9J3
Tel.: +1 613 745 2665
Fax: +1 613 745 7660
E-mail: renouf@fox.nstn.ca
Website: www.renoufbooks.com

• CHILE
Librería - Oficina Regional, FAO
c/o FAO, Oficina Regional para América
Latina y el Caribe (RLC)
Avda. Dag Hammarskjold, 3241
Vitacura, Santiago
Tel.: +56 2 33 72 314
Correo electrónico:
german.rojas@field.fao.org
Universitaria Textolibros Ltda.
Avda. L. Bernardo O'Higgins 1050
Santiago

• CHINA
China National Publications
Import & Export Corporation
16 Gongti East Road, Beijing 100020
Tel.: +86 10 6506 3070
Fax: +86 10 6506 3101
E-mail: serials@cnpiec.com.cn

• COLOMBIA
INFOENLACE LTDA
Calle 72 Nº 13-23 Piso 3
Edificio Nueva Granada
Santafé de Bogotá
Tel.: 2558783-2557969
Fax: 2480808-2176435
Correo electrónico:
infoenlace@gaitana.interred.net.co

• CONGO
Office national des librairies
populaires
B.P. 577, Brazzaville

• COSTA RICA
Librería Lehmann S.A.
Av. Central, Apartado 10011
1000 San José
CINDE
Coalición Costarricense de Iniciativas
de Desarrollo
Apartado 7170, 1000 San José
Correo electrónico:
rtacinde@sol.rassa.co.cr

• CÔTE D'IVOIRE
CEDA
04 B.P. 541, Abidjan 04
Tél.: +225 22 20 55
Télécopie: +225 21 72 62

• CUBA
Ediciones Cubanas
Empresa de Comercio Exterior
de Publicaciones
Obispo 461, Apartado 605, La Habana

• CZECH REPUBLIC
Artia Pegas Press Ltd
Import of Periodicals
Palác Metro, PO Box 825
Národní 25, 111 21 Praha 1

• DENMARK
Munksgaard, Direct
Ostergate 26 A - Postbox 173
DK - 1005 Copenhagen K.
Tel.: +45 331 28570
Fax: +45 331 29387
E-mail: direct@munksgaarddirect.dk
URL: www.munksgaardirect.dk

• REPÚBLICA DOMINICANA
CUESTA - Centro del libro
Av. 27 de Febrero, esq. A. Lincoln
Centro Comercial Nacional
Apartado 1241, Santo Domingo
CEDAF - Centro para el Desarrollo
Agropecuario y Forestal, Inc.
Calle José Amado Soler, 50 - Urban.
Paraíso
Apartado Postal, 567-2, Santo Domingo
Tel.: +001 809 544-0616/544-0634/
565-5603
Fax: +001 809 544-4727/567-6989
Correo electrónico: fda@Codetel.net.do

• ECUADOR
Libri Mundi, Librería Internacional
Juan León Mera 851
Apartado Postal 3029, Quito
Correo electrónico:
librimul@librimundi.com.ec
Universidad Agraria del Ecuador
Centro de Información Agraria
Av. 23 de julio, Apartado 09-01-1248
Guayaquil
Librería Española
Murgeón 364 y Ulloa, Quito

• EGYPT
MERIC
The Middle East Readers' Information
Centre
2 Baghat Aly Street, Appt. 24
El Masry Tower D
Cairo/Zamalek
E-mail: mafouda@meric-co.com
Tel.: +202 3413824; +202 34038818
Fax: +202 3419355

• ESPAÑA
Librería Agrícola
Fernando VI 2, 28004 Madrid
Librería de la Generalitat
de Catalunya
Rambla dels Estudis 118 (Palau Moja)
08002 Barcelona
Tel.: +34 93 302 6462
Fax: +34 93 302 1299
Mundi Prensa Libros S.A.
Castelló 37, 28001 Madrid
Tel.: +34 914 36 37 00
Fax: +34 915 75 39 98
Sitio Web: www.mundiprensa.com
Correo electrónico:
libreria@mundiprensa.es
Mundi Prensa - Barcelona
Consejo de Ciento 391
08009 Barcelona
Tel.: +34 934 88 34 92
Fax: +34 934 87 76 59

• FINLAND
Akateeminen Kirjakauppa
Subscription Services
PO Box 23, FIN-00371 Helsinki
Tel.: +358 9 121 4416
Fax: +358 9 121 4450

• FRANCE
Editions A. Pedone
13, rue Soufflot, 75005 Paris
Lavoisier Tec & Doc
14, rue de Provigny
94236 Cachan Cedex
Mél.: livres@lavoisier.fr
Site Web: www.lavoisier.fr
Librairie du commerce international
10, avenue d'Iéna
75783 Paris Cedex 16
Mél.: pl@net-export.fr
Site Web: www.cfce.fr
WORLD DATA
10, rue Nicolas Flamand
75004 Paris
Tél.: +33 1 4278 0578
Télécopie: +33 1 4278 1472

• GERMANY
Alexander Horn Internationale
Buchhandlung
Friedrichstrasse 34
D-65185 Wiesbaden
Tel.: +49 6121 37 42 12
S. Toeche-Mittler GmbH
Versandbuchhandlung
Hindenburgstrasse 33
D-64295 Darmstadt
Tel.: +49 6151 336 65
Fax: +49 6151 314 043
E-mail: triops@booksell.com
Website: www.booksell.com/triops
Uno Verlag
Poppelsdorfer Allee 55
D-53115 Bonn 1
Tel.: +49 228 94 90 20
Fax: +49 228 21 74 92
E-mail: unoverlag@aol.com
Website: www.uno-verlag.de

• GHANA
SEDCO Publishing Ltd
Sedco House, Tabon Street
Off Ring Road Central, North Ridge
PO Box 2051, Accra
Readwide Bookshop Ltd
PO Box 0600 Osu, Accra
Tel.: +233 21 22 1387
Fax: +233 2166 3347
E-mail: readwide@africaonline.cpm.gh

• GREECE
Papasotiriou S.A.
35 Stournara Str., 10682 Athens
Tel.: +30 1 3302 980
Fax: +30 1 3648254

• GUYANA
Guyana National Trading
Corporation Ltd
45-47 Water Street, PO Box 308
Georgetown

• HONDURAS
Escuela Agrícola Panamericana
Librería RTAC
El Zamorano, Apartado 93, Tegucigalpa
Oficina de la Escuela Agrícola
Panamericana en Tegucigalpa
Blvd. Morazán, Apts. Glapson
Apartado 93, Tegucigalpa

• HUNGARY
Librotrade Kft.
PO Box 126, H-1656 Budapest
Tel.: +36 1 256 1672
Fax: +36 1 256 8727

• INDIA
Allied Publisher Ltd
751 Mount Road
Chennai 600 002
Tel.: +91 44 8523938/8523984
Fax: +91 44 8520649
E-mail:
allied.mds@smb.sprintrpg.ems.vsnl.net.in
EWP Affiliated East-West
Press PVT, Ltd
G-I/16, Ansari Road, Darya Ganj
New Delhi 110 002
Tel.: +91 11 3264 180
Fax: +91 11 3260 358
E-mail: affiliat@nda.vsnl.net.in
Oxford Book and Stationery Co.
Scindia House
New Delhi 110001
Tel.: +91 113315310
Fax: +91 113713275
E-mail: oxford@vsnl.com
Periodical Expert Book Agency
G-56, 2nd Floor, Laxmi Nagar
Vikas Marg, Delhi 110092
Tel: +91 11 2215045/2150534
Fax: +91 11 2418599
E-mail: oriental@nde.vsnl.net.in
Bookwell
Head Office:
2/72, Nirankari Colony, New Delhi - 110009
Tel.: +91 11 725 1283
Fax: +91 11 328 13 15
Sales Office:
24/4800, Ansari Road
Darya Ganj, New Delhi - 110002
Tel.: +91 11 326 8786
E-mail: bkwell@nde.vsnl.net.in

• IRAN
The FAO Bureau, International
and Regional Specialized
Organizations Affairs
Ministry of Agriculture of the Islamic
Republic of Iran
Keshavarz Bld, M.O.A., 17th floor
Teheran

• IRELAND
Office of Public Work
4-5 Harcourt Road, Dublin 2

• ISRAEL
R.O.Y. International
PO Box 13056, Tel Aviv 61130
E-mail: royil@netvision.net.il

• ITALY
FAO Bookshop
Viale delle Terme di Caracalla
00100 Roma
Tel.: +39 06 5705 2313
Fax: +39 06 5705 3360
E-mail: publications-sales@fao.org

WHERE TO PURCHASE FAO PUBLICATIONS LOCALLY
POINTS DE VENTE DES PUBLICATIONS DE LA FAO
PUNTOS DE VENTA DE PUBLICACIONES DE LA FAO

Libreria Commissionaria Sansoni
S.p.A. - Licosa
Via Duca di Calabria 1/1
50125 Firenze
Tel.: + 39 55 64 8 31
Fax: +39 55 64 12 57
E-mail: licosa@ftbcc.it
Libreria Scientifica Dott. Lucio de
Biasio "Aeiou"
Via Coronelli 6, 20146 Milano

• **JAPAN**
Far Eastern Booksellers
(Kyokuto Shoten Ltd)
12 Kanda-Jimbocho 2 chome
Chiyoda-ku - PO Box 72
Tokyo 101-91
Tel.: +81 3 3265 7531
Fax: +81 3 3265 4656
Maruzen Company Ltd
PO Box 5050
Tokyo International 100-31
Tel.: +81 3 3275 8585
Fax: +81 3 3275 0656
E-mail: h_sugiyama@maruzen.co.jp

• **KENYA**
Text Book Centre Ltd
Kijabe Street
PO Box 47540, Nairobi
Tel.: +254 2 330 342
Fax: +254 2 22 57 79
Inter Africa Book Distribution
Kencom House, Moi Avenue
PO Box 73580, Nairobi
Tel.: +254 2 211 184
Fax: +254 2 22 3 5 70
Legacy Books
Mezzanine 1, Loita House, Loita Street
Nairobi, PO Box 68077
Tel.: +254 2 303853
Fax: +254 2 330854

• **LUXEMBOURG**
M.J. De Lannoy
202, avenue du Roi
B-1060, Bruxelles (Belgique)
Mél.: jean.de.lannoy@infoboard.be

• **MADAGASCAR**
Centre d'Information et de
Documentation Scientifique et
Technique
Ministère de la recherche appliquée
au développement
B.P. 6224, Tsimbazaza, Antananarivo

• **MALAYSIA**
Southbound
Suite 20F Northam House
55 Jalan Sultan Ahmad Shah
10050 Penang
E-mail: chin@south.pc.my
URL: www.southbound.com.my
Tel.: +60 4 2282169
Fax: +60 4 2281758

• **MALI**
Librairie Traore
Rue Soundiata Keita X 115
B.P. 3243, Bamako

• **MAROC**
La Librairie Internationale
70, rue T'ssoule
B.P. 302 (RP), Rabat
Tél./Télécopie: 212 7 75 01 83

• **MÉXICO**
Librería, Universidad Autónoma de
Chapingo
56230 Chapingo
Libros y Editoriales S.A.
Av. Progreso Nº 202-1º Piso A
Apartado. Postal 18922
Col. Escandón, 11800 México D.F.
Mundi Prensa Mexico, S.A.
Río Pánuco, 141 Col. Cuauhtémoc
C.P. 06500, México, DF
Tel.: +52 5 533 56 58
Fax: +52 5 514 67 99
Correo electrónico:
1015452361@compuserve.com

• **NETHERLANDS**
Roodveldt Import b.v.
Brouwersgracht 288
1013 HG Amsterdam
Tel.: +31 20 622 80 35
Fax: +31 20 625 54 93
E-mail: roodboek@euronet.nl
Swets & Zeitlinger b.v.
PO Box 830, 2160 Lisse
Heereweg 347 B, 2161 CA Lisse
E-mail: infono@swets.nl
Website: www.swets.nl

• **NEW ZEALAND**
Legislation Services
PO Box 12418
Thorndon, Wellington
E-mail: gppmjxf@gp.co.nz
Oasis Official
PO Box 3627, Wellington
Tel.: +64 4 499 1551
Fax: +64 4 499 1972
E-mail: oasis@clear.net.nz
Website: www.oasisbooks.co.nzl

• **NICARAGUA**
Librería HISPAMER
Costado Este Univ. Centroamericana
Apartado Postal A-221, Managua

• **NIGERIA**
University Bookshop (Nigeria) Ltd
University of Ibadan, Ibadan

• **PAKISTAN**
Mirza Book Agency
65 Shahrah-e-Quaid-e-Azam
PO Box 729, Lahore 3

• **PARAGUAY**
Librería Intercontinental
Editora e Impresora S.R.L.
Caballero 270 c/Mcal Estigarribia
Asunción

• **PERÚ**
INDEAR
Jirón Apurímac 375, Casilla 4937
Lima 1
Universidad Nacional «Pedro Ruiz
Gallo»
Facultad de Agronomía, A.P. 795
Lambayeque (Chiclayo)

• **PHILIPPINES**
International Booksource Center, Inc.
1127-A Antipolo St., Barangay Valenzuela
Makati City
Tel.: +632 8966501/8966505/8966507
Fax: +632 8966497
E-mail: ibcdina@webquest.com

• **POLAND**
Ars Polona
Krakowskie Przedmiescie 7
00-950 Warsaw

• **PORTUGAL**
Livraria Portugal, Dias e Andrade
Ltda.
Rua do Carmo, 70-74
Apartado 2681, 1200 Lisboa Codex

• **SINGAPORE**
Select Books Pte Ltd
03-15 Tanglin Shopping Centre
19 Tanglin Road, Singapore 1024
Tel.: +65 732 1515
Fax: +65 736 0855

• **SLOVAK REPUBLIC**
Institute of Scientific and Technical
Information for Agriculture
Samova 9, 950 10 Nitra
Tel.: +421 87 522 185
Fax: +421 87 525 275
E-mail: uvtip@nr.sanet.sk

• **SOMALIA**
Samater
PO Box 936, Mogadishu

• **SOUTH AFRICA**
David Philip Publishers (Pty) Ltd
PO Box 23408, Claremont 7735
Tel.: Cape Town +27 21 64 4136
Fax: Cape Town+ 27 21 64 3358
E-mail: dpp@iafrica.com
Website: www.twisted.co.za

• **SRI LANKA**
M.D. Gunasena & Co. Ltd
217 Olcott Mawatha, PO Box 246
Colombo 11

• **SUISSE**
UN Bookshop
Palais des Nations
CH-1211 Genève 1
Site Web: www.un.org
Van Diermen Editions Techniques
ADECO
41 Lacuez, CH-1807 Blonzy

• **SURINAME**
Vaco n.v. in Suriname
Domineestraat 26, PO Box 1841
Paramaribo

• **SWEDEN**
Wennergren Williams AB
PO Box 1305, S-171 25 Solna
Tel.: +46 8 705 9750
Fax: +46 8 27 00 71
E-mail: mail@wwi.se
Bokdistributören
c/o Longus Books Import
PO Box 610, S-151 27 Södertälje
Tel.: +46 8 55 09 49 70
Fax: +46 55 01 76 10; E-mail:
lis.ledin@hk.akademibokhandeln.se

• **THAILAND**
Suksapan Panit
Mansion 9, Rajdamnern Avenue, Bangkok

• **TOGO**
Librairie du Bon Pasteur
B.P. 1164, Lomé

• **TUNISIE**
Société tunisienne de diffusion
5, avenue de Carthage, Tunis

• **TURKEY**
DUNYA INFOTEL
100. Yil Mahallesi
34440 Bagcilar, Istanbul
Tel.: +90 212 629 0808
Fax: +90 212 629 4689
E-mail: dunya@dunya-gazete.com.tr
Website: www.dunya.com

• **UGANDA**
Fountain Publishers Ltd
PO Box 488, Kampala
Tel.: +256 41 259 163
Fax: +256 41 251 160

• **UNITED KINGDOM**
The Stationery Office
51 Nine Elms Lane
London SW8 5DR
Tel.: +44 171 873 9090 (orders)
+44 171 873 0011 (inquiries)
Fax: + 44 171 873 8463
and through The Stationery Office
Bookshops
E-mail: postmaster@theso.co.uk
Website: www.the-stationery-office.co.uk
Electronic products only:
Microinfo Ltd
PO Box 3, Omega Road
Alton, Hampshire GU34 2PG
Tel.: +44 1420 86 848
Fax: +44 1420 89 889
E-mail: emedia@microinfo.co.uk
Website: www.microinfo.co.uk
Intermediate Technology Bookshop
103-105 Southampton Row
London WC1B 4HH
Tel.: +44 171 436 9761
Fax: +44 171 436 2013
E-mail: orders@itpubs.org.uk
Website: www.oneworld.org/itdg/
publications.html

• **UNITED STATES**
Publications:
BERNAN Associates (ex UNIPUB)
4611/F Assembly Drive
Lanham, MD 20706-4391
Toll-free: +1800 274 4447
Fax: +1 800 865 3450
E-mail: query@bernan.com
Website: www.bernan.com
United Nations Publications
Two UN Plaza, Room DC2-853
New York, NY 10017
Tel.: 212-963-8302 or 800-253-9646
Fax: 212-963-3489
E-mail: publications@un.org
Website: www.unog.ch
UN Bookshop (direct sales)
The United Nations Bookshop
General Assembly Building Room 32
New York, NY 10017
Tel.: +1 212 963 7680
Fax: +1 212 963 4910
E-mail: bookshop@un.org
Website: www.un.org
Periodicals:
Ebsco Subscription Services
PO Box 1943
Birmingham, AL 35201-1943
Tel.: +1 205 991 6600
Fax: +1 205 991 1449
The Faxon Company Inc.
15 Southwest Park
Westwood, MA 02090
Tel.: 6117-329-3350
Telex: 95-1980
Cable: FW Faxon Wood

• **URUGUAY**
Librería Agropecuaria S.R.L.
Buenos Aires 335, Casilla 1755
Montevideo C.P. 11000

• **VENEZUELA**
Fundación La Era Agrícola
Calle 31 Junín Qta Coromoto 5-49
Apartado 456, Mérida
Fudeco, Librería
Avenida Libertador-Este
Ed. Fudeco, Apartado 254
Barquisimeto C.P. 3002, Ed. Lara
Tel.: +58 51 538 022
Fax: +58 51 544 394
Librería FAGRO
Universidad Central de Venezuela (UCV)
Maracay
Librería Universitaria, C.A.
Av. 3, entre Calles 29 y 30
Nº 29-25 Edif. EVA, Mérida
Fax: +58 74 52 0956
Tamanaco Libros Técnicos S.R.L.
Centro Comercial Ciudad Tamanaco
Nivel C-2, Caracas
Tel.: +58 2 261 3344/261 3335
Tecni-Ciencia Libros S.A.
Torre Phelps-Mezzanina
Plaza Venezuela
Apartado Postal: 20.315, 1020 Caracas
Tel.: +58 2 782 8698/781 9945
Correo electrónico: tchlibros@ibm.net

• **ZIMBABWE**
Grassroots Books
The Book Café
Fife Avenue, Harare;
61a Fort Street, Bulawayo
Tel.: +263 4 79 31 82
Fax: +263 4 72 62 43